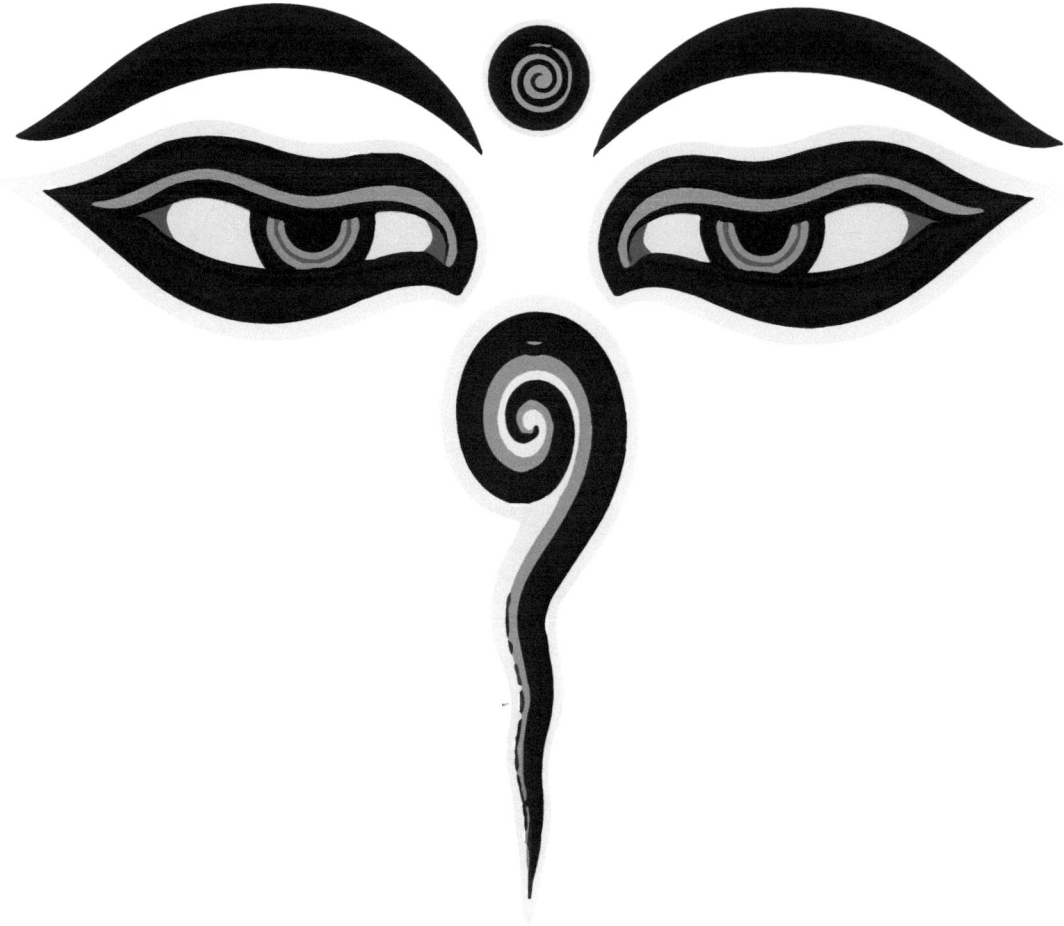

Preface

After 10 years of teaching and professional studies and more than twenty years of practice, the time has come to write something down. A good friend's first words were: "oh how pretentious!". I totally agree. Who am I to think I have something worthy to contribute to the antiquity of yoga? Who am I to stand alongside masters like Patanjali, Bodhidharma, Gautama Buddha, Jesus, Satchidananda, Iyengar, Sivananda, Ramana Maharishi, Yogananda, Pattabhi Jois or Ramakrishna, and assume my words, practice and knowledge are relevant? Like these men, I am one of spiritual integrity but unlike them, I am alive, and therefore take it as my duty to share my truth with others.

I write this book to share what I have learnt through my years of practice and study. I do not say that my own practice and my relationship with God is better than anybody else's, for that is a matter between them and God. Nevertheless, like those men before me, I share my truth with others as it has been the custom for thousands of years and which shall continue long after my time.

The book you are holding is my humble attempt to express and interpret the ancient oral tradition of yoga. There is no new information, only a contemporary interpretation of the truth. The world changes but the human's soul remains the same, it is constant, infinite like God or Mother Nature. The stories repeat and are told over and over to generations anew, each make of it what they will, according to their environment. Some comprehend the divine reality rejoicing in it while others may fear it. Though the truth is often concealed it is very much alive. This book is a guide that provides you with tools to help on your self-discovery journey and spiritual awakening. Understanding Yoga and how the body responds to it is the key to a happy life. That said, I'd like to thank my students as without them there is no teacher, no class and no continuity.

Thank you for those whose contributions made this book happen; from the Chai Wallah to the electric company, from the photographer to the garbage man, although you don't know it, you have all helped immensely. And that means you too, the reader. I hope that by reading this book and thinking about some of the proposed concepts you'll discover the magic for yourself. It really is that simple. I sincerely hope this book helps you in your yogic explorations.

Namaste

Wolfy 2019

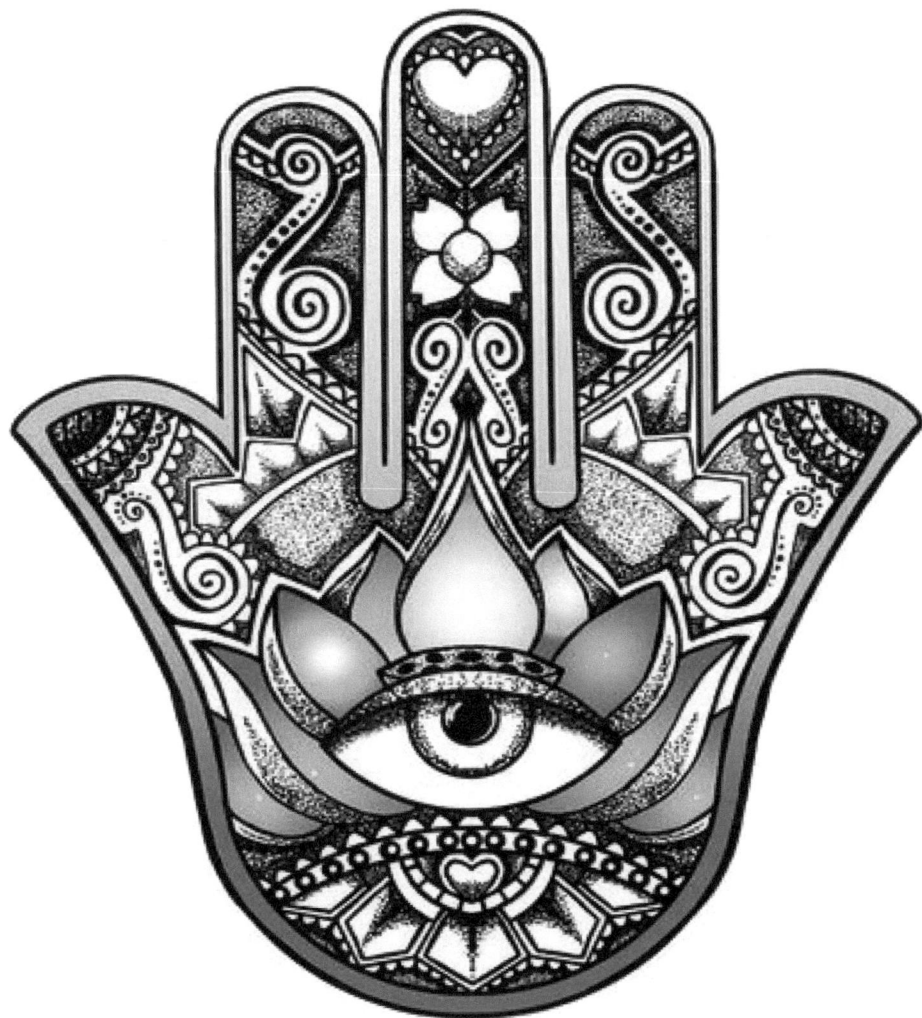

For my father,
who taught me to be a man
and for my mother,
who taught me to be
a gentle man.

Hey friends! Salaam alaikum (may peace be upon you).

Welcome to the wonderful world of yoga.
My name is Wolfy and I will be your guide and humble narrator as we journey into the basics of yoga.

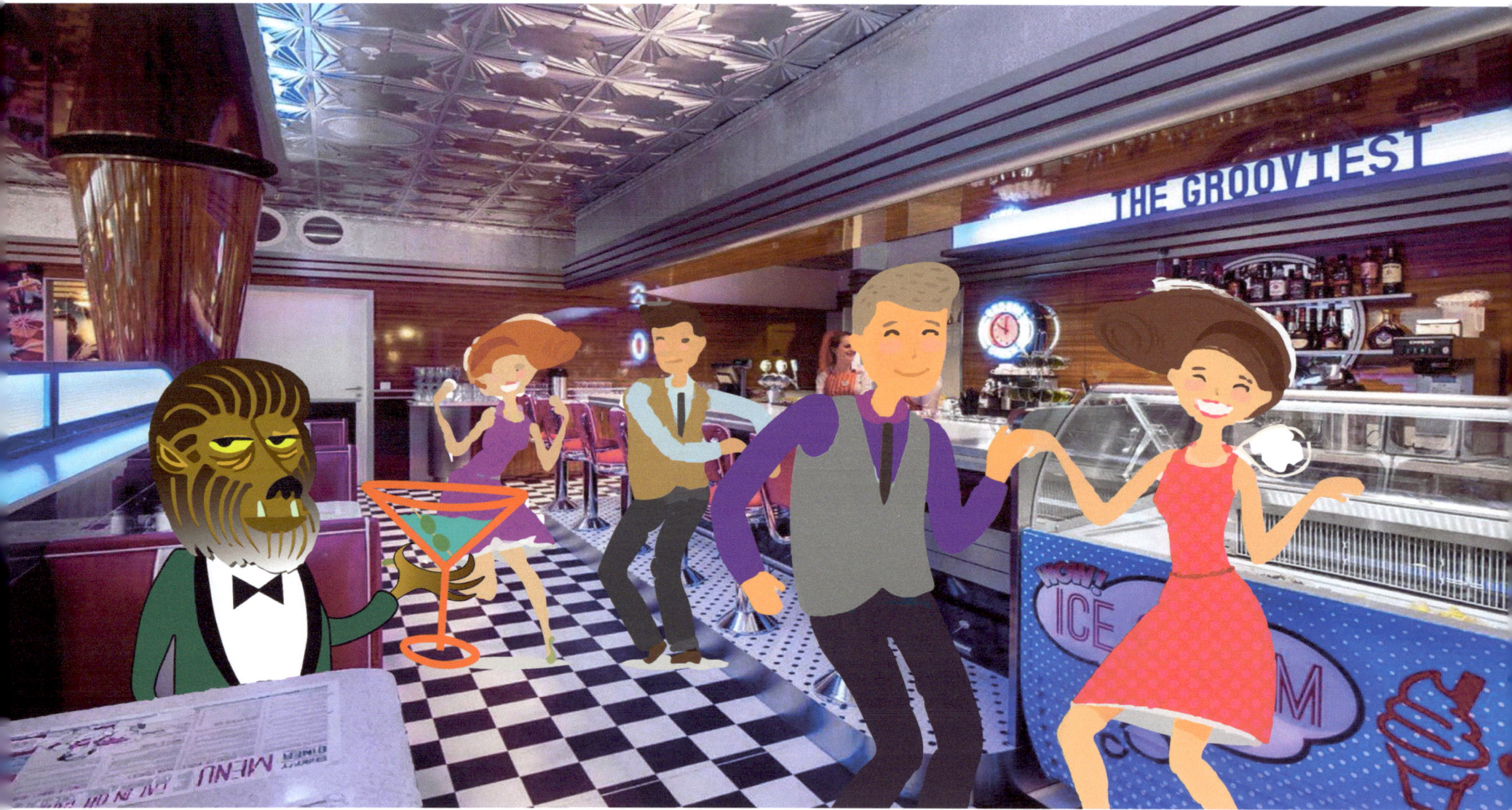

Now you're probably wondering what we're doing here at The Grooviest Scoop? Well it's one of my fave hangouts; a real gone swingin' shindig! I'm nuts for a good time and im partial to the odd martini too, but thats not yoga. Yoga is an inward journey, away from the ego, to the centre of who you really are. If we're going to practice yoga it means we will look for and try to understand this centre.

Sometimes we need to be loud and outrageous and expend large amounts of energy. At other times we need to be quiet, listen to our inner voice and tap into more subtle energies. This is all part of living. As we get older we notice the cycles of life; sometimes you're up, sometimes you're down, sometimes its hot, sometimes cold, sometimes you're angry and at other times you're happy, sometimes you're hungry and sometimes not . . . And round and round it goes.

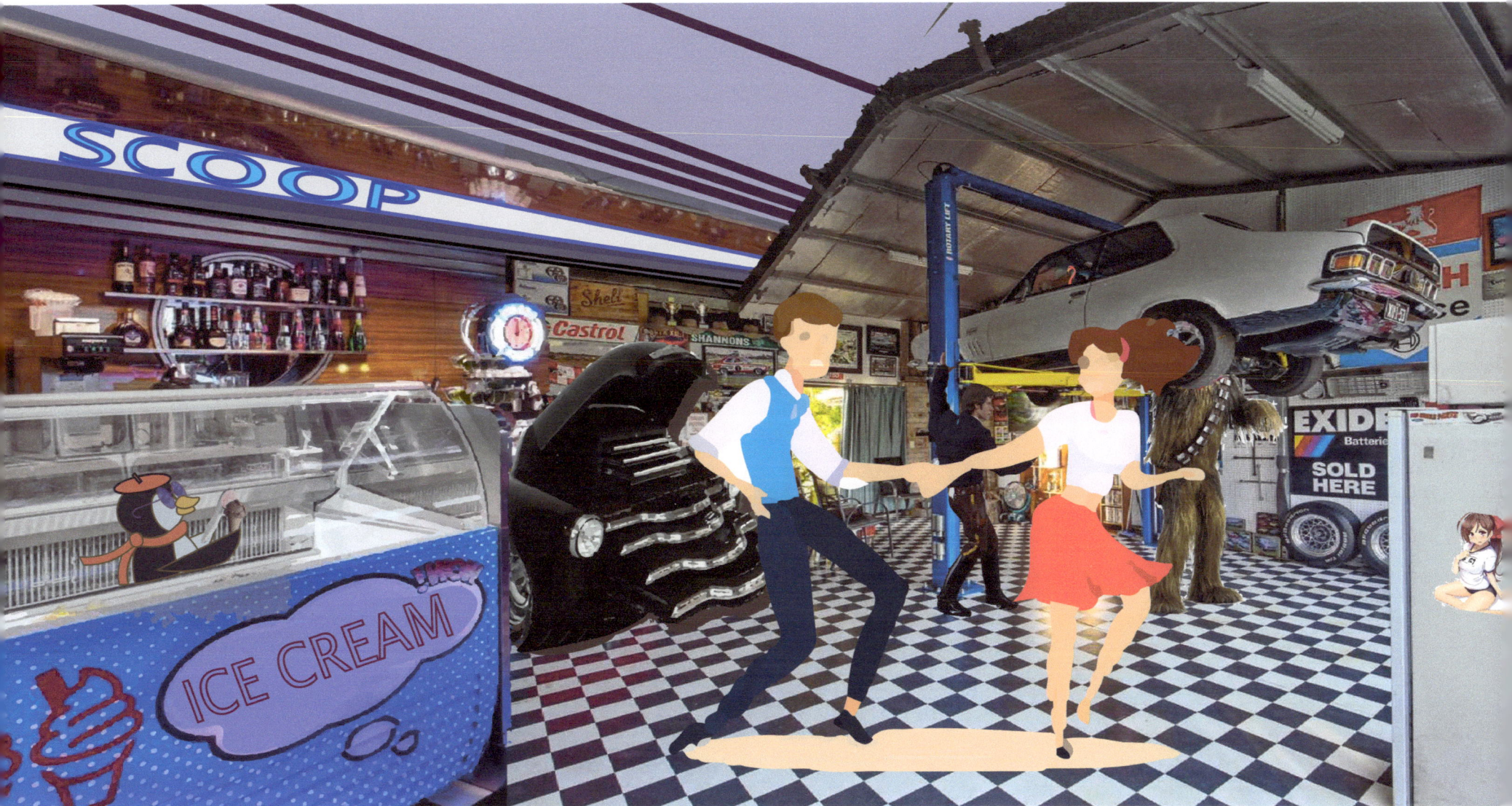

I've spent my whole life traveling the world, studying the dynamics of human movement and how it manifests in different cultures. From my understanding I believe that yoga best describes the fundamentals of human life. If you move your body, breathe and are conscious of what you're doing, you're doing yoga. It's that simple. People will call it other names but it's all yoga.

You probably already have an idea in your mind of what yoga is but I suggest you throw it away. Delete it from your mind as it is usually a contrived media image, not even close to the real thing. Cast your mind for a moment to the old bastion of the Christian world - Christmas. For all it is worth this day no longer celebrates Jesus' birthday as originally intended. It has become a cesspit of market and media driven propaganda designed to promote consumerism.

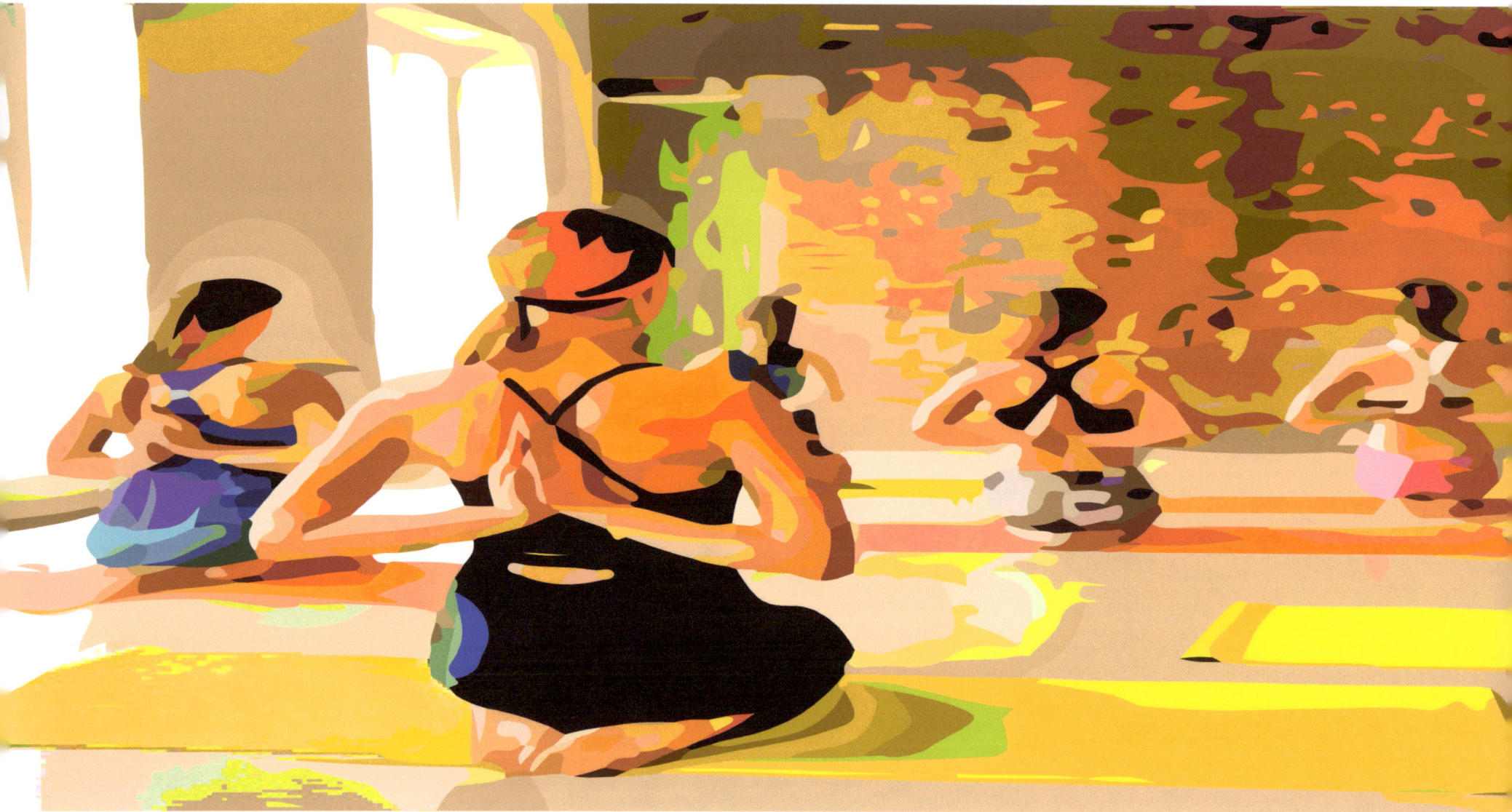

It is the same with Easter, Valentine's day, Mother's day, Father's day and many others traditionally celebrated by western society. It saddens my heart to say that yoga is not safe from this evil force either, it is saturated with selfish devils masquerading as enlightened gurus ready to take your money. Once these scoundrels see there is a dollar to be made, they grab the cash cow and milk it for all its worth, until it becomes a polished shrine to the celebration of stupidity that we salute year after year. Just like Christmas.

Another point to consider is the abuse of power. Devious people in positions of power often take advantage of beginner's vulnerability leading them into a dark world of manipulation and degradation. Financial and sexual abuse are common. I shouldn't have to mention the Catholic priests, Yoga gurus or movie directors as their actions hold enough notoriety and speak for themselves. The more you look, the more greed and selfishness you'll find.

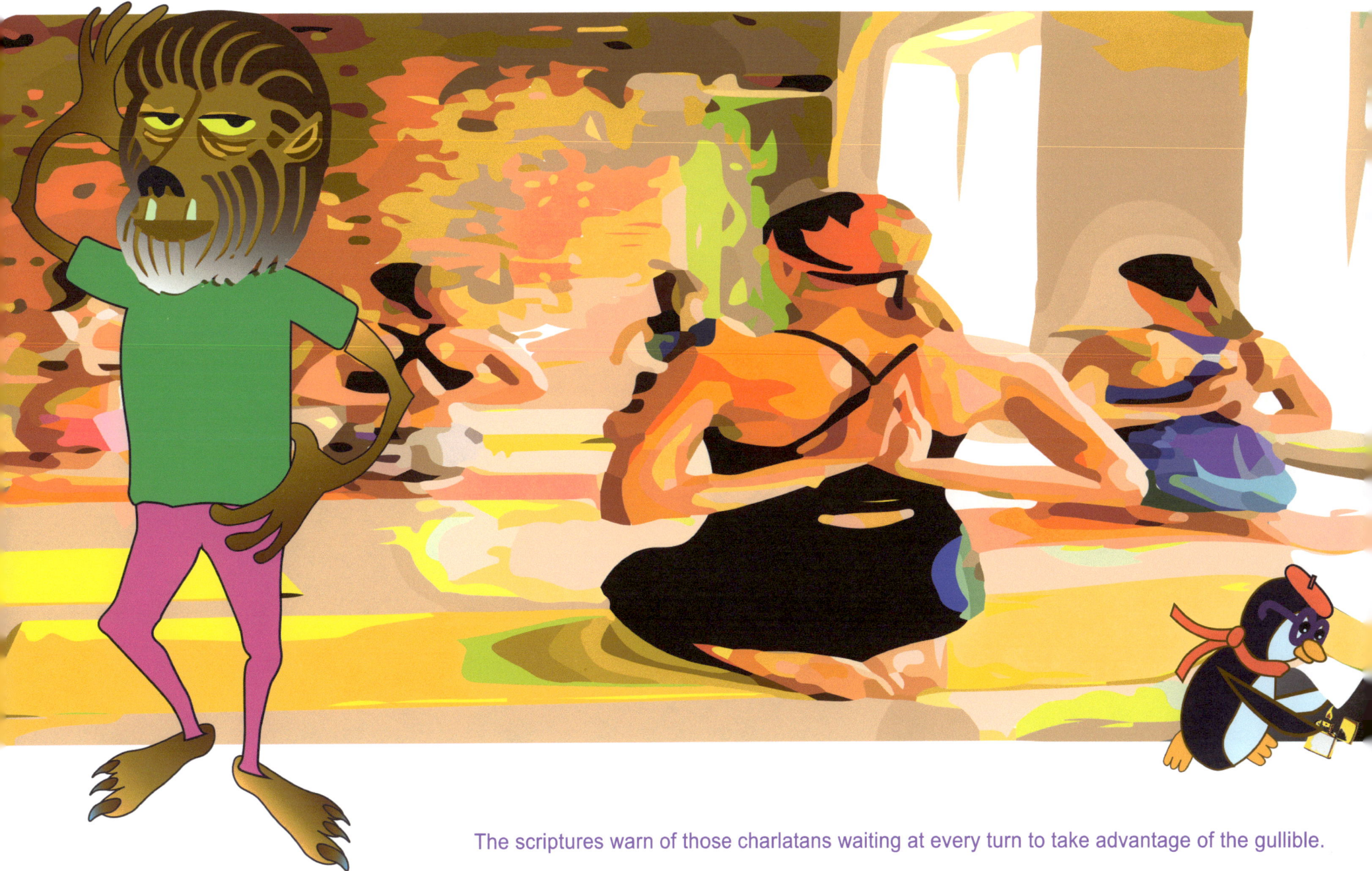

The scriptures warn of those charlatans waiting at every turn to take advantage of the gullible.

Oh my brothers and sisters beware, be very aware! Be on guard for those silver tongued rogues you give your mind and body to, for they do not care for it the way you do. They seek to exploit your vulnerability and they always come at a price. They will selfishly use your lack of knowledge against you and call it healing.

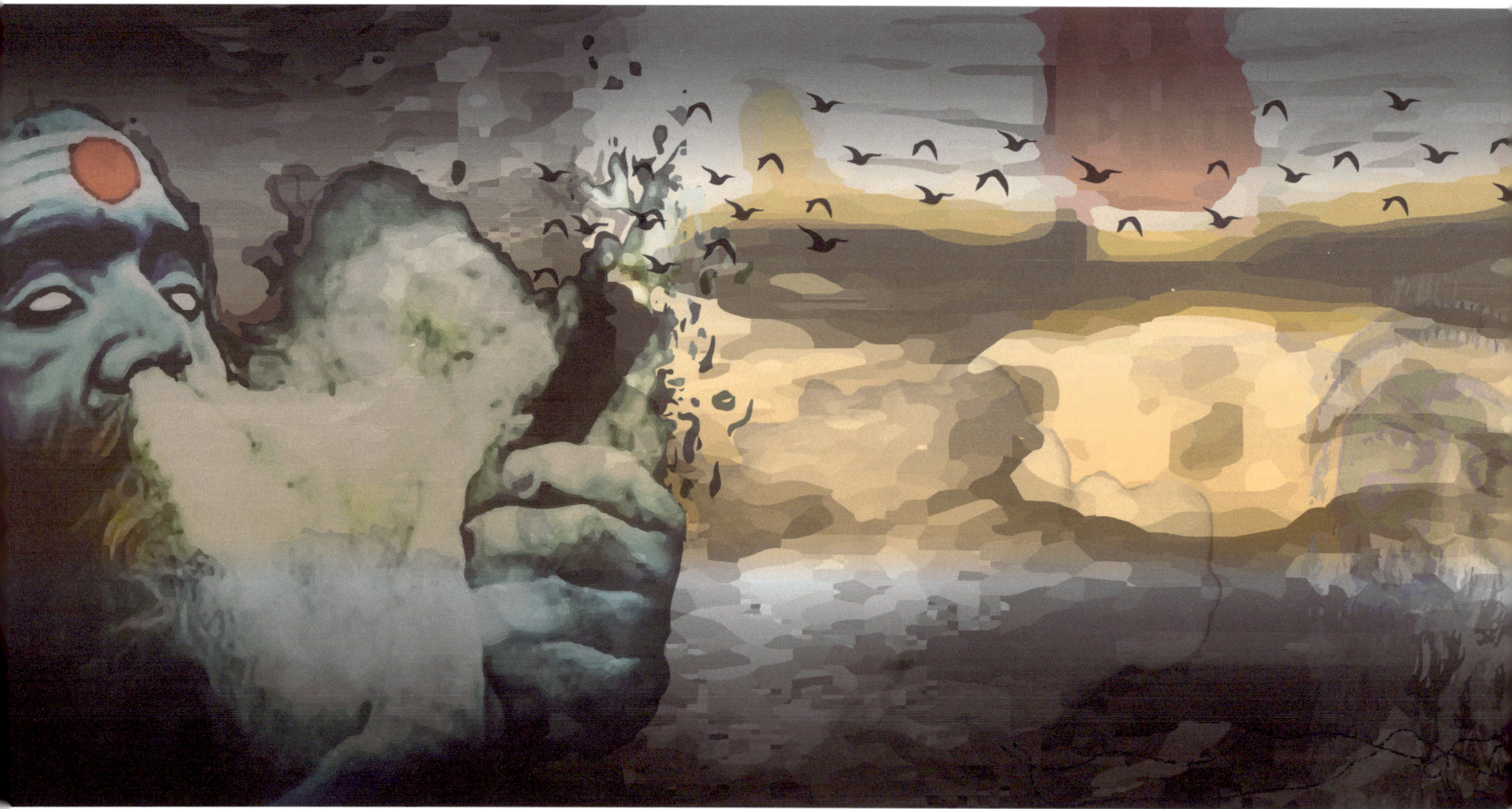

We see this kind of behaviour flourishing now as the sickness industry. People are on their deathbed and still the healers ask for more money, just like kicking a dog when it is hurt. But enough of these debaucherous tales, we are here to talk about healing, not stealing!
The warning has been given.

As the great Buddha says, 'doubt everything and find your own light'. Live your life and discover what is truth for you, not what is truth for others. I will say the same. Read this book or better still have someone read it to you, practice the techniques and have fun, make up your own mind if it works or not.

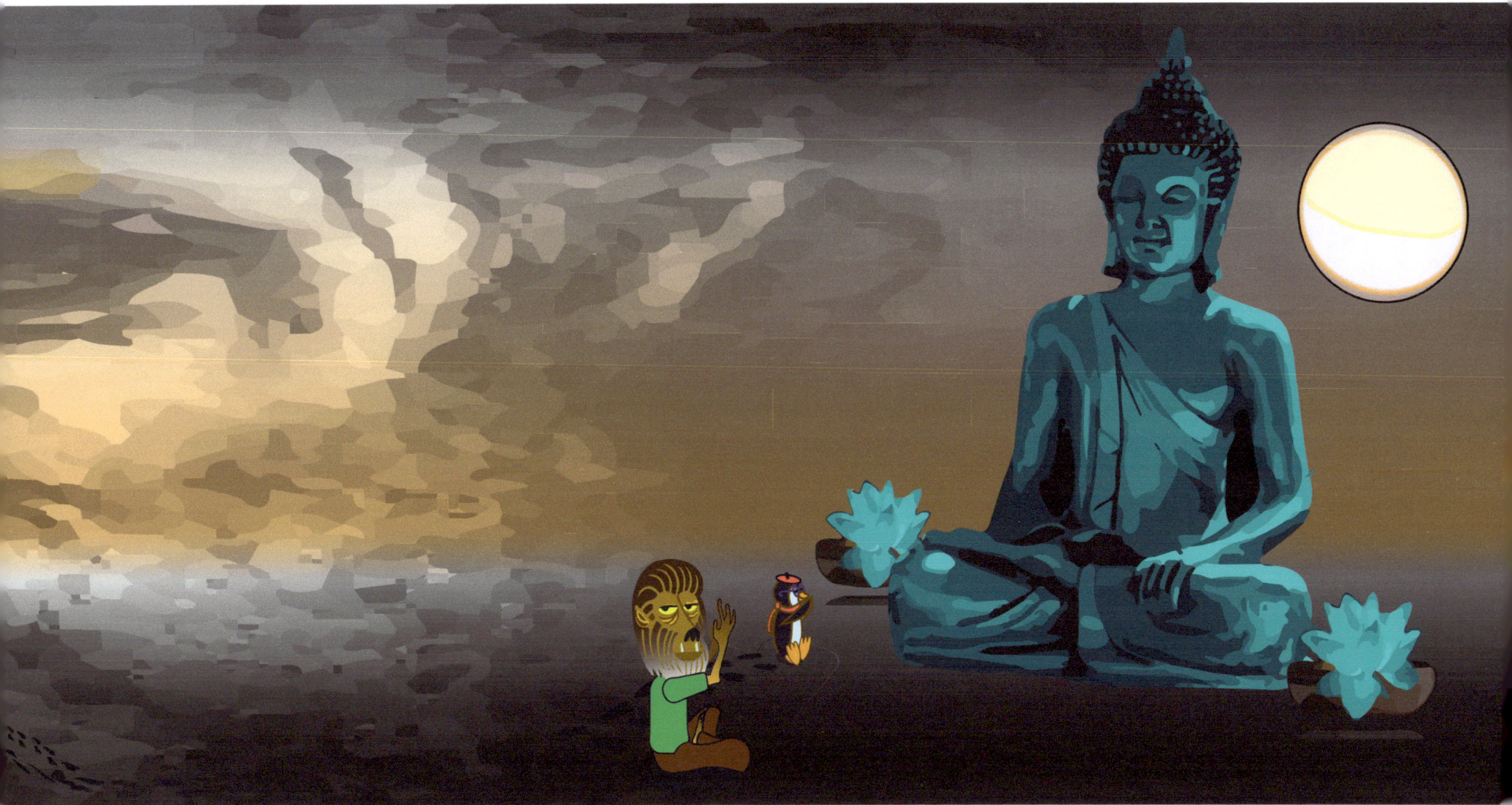

Here, take my hand and let us begin our adventure.
You can thank me later.
My buddy Pengu wants to come too.

The origins of any great philosophy are often hard to identify. Yogic philosophy is no different. The Yoga Sutras as expounded by the great sage Patanjali, circa 300 – 400 AD, comprise the first and foremost scripture of yoga. For thousands of years before this yoga was an oral tradition handed down from teacher to disciple. There is no new information, just a retelling of the story. All variations of yoga are adaptations of Patanjali's Yoga Sutras and no serious study would be complete without a thorough inquiry and consideration of these sutras.

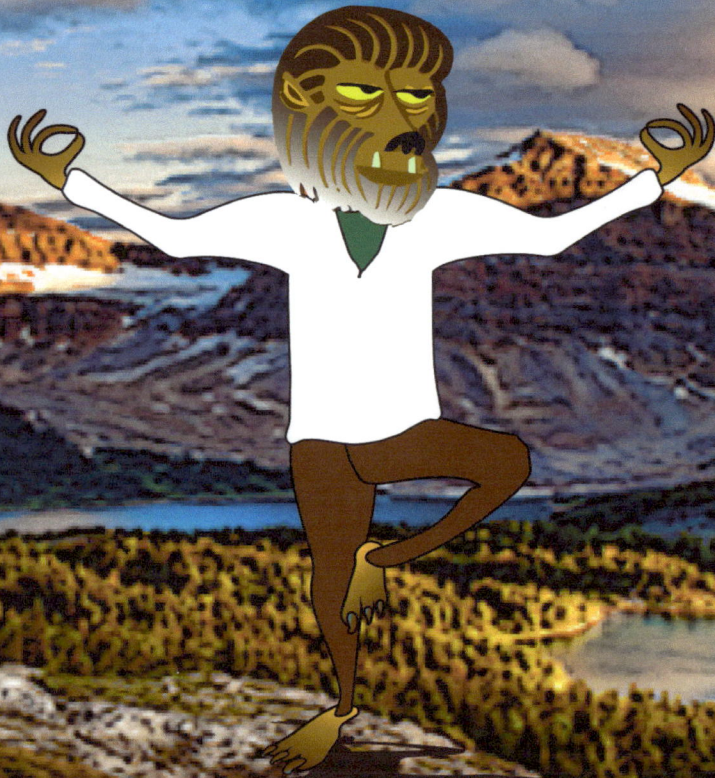

Yoga is the search for truth; the truth or science of the human body. It is a complete approach that covers every aspect of being human.

To quote the great sage Satchidananda;

"Yoga does not simply advocate meditation and posture but takes into consideration the entire life of a person. Its philosophy is scientific. It welcomes and in fact demands experimental verification by the student. Its ultimate aim is to bring about a thorough metamorphosis of the individual who practices it sincerely. Its goal is nothing less than the total transformation of a seemingly limited physical, mental and emotional person into a fully illuminated, thoroughly harmonized and perfected being – from an individual with likes and dislikes, pains and pleasures, successes and failures, to a sage of permanent peace, joy and selfless dedication to the entire creation."

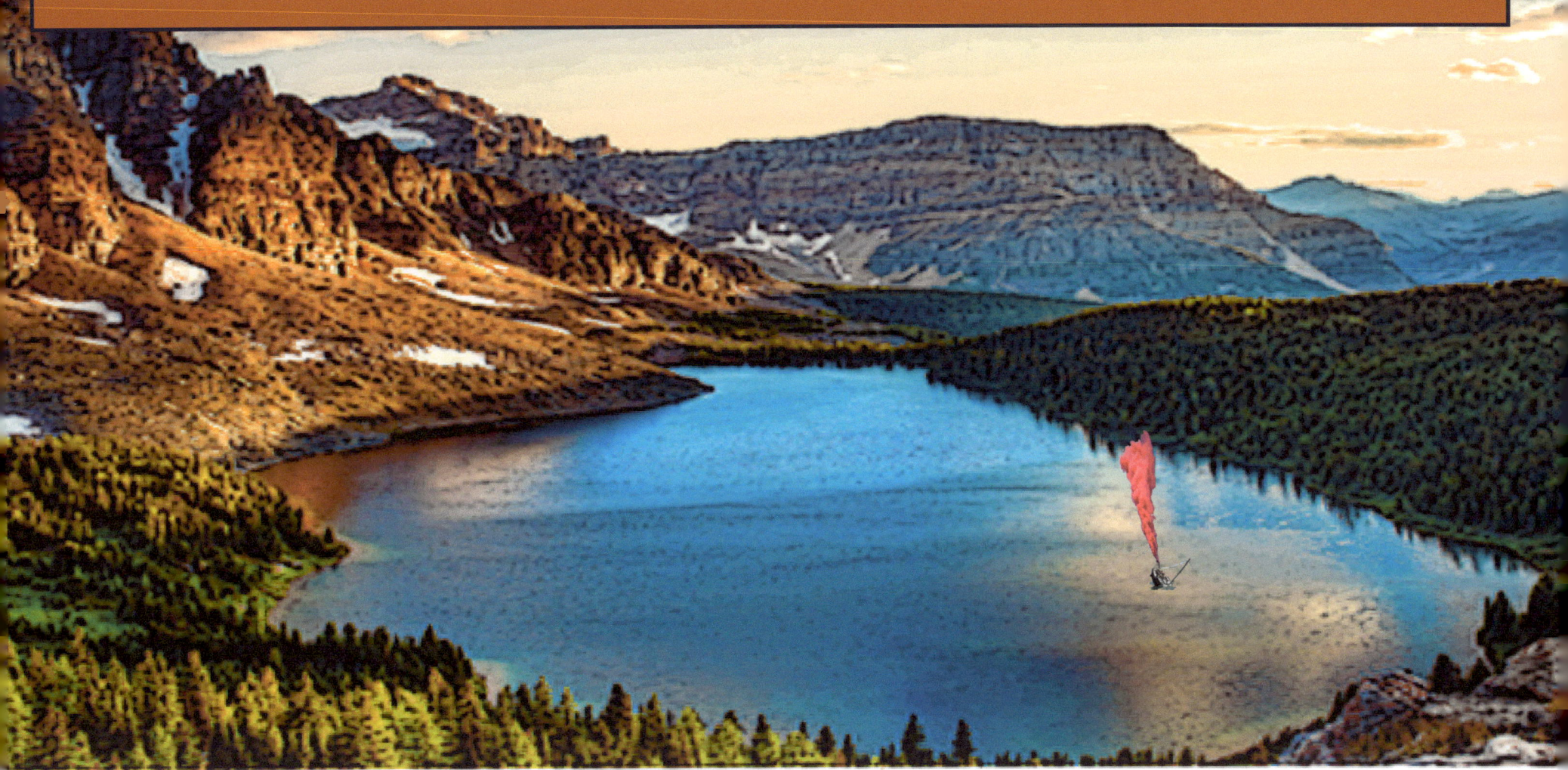

Wow, now that was an inspiring statement! Thanks Satchi.
Take a moment to read it again and let it sink in.

This is the very core of yoga; a metamorphosis. And each great transformation takes time. Just like a caterpillar into a butterfly, a tree into a table, a boy into a man. It may sound lofty but I ask you to try it for yourself and see if it works for you. Some results will be immediate, others will take years to come to fruition.

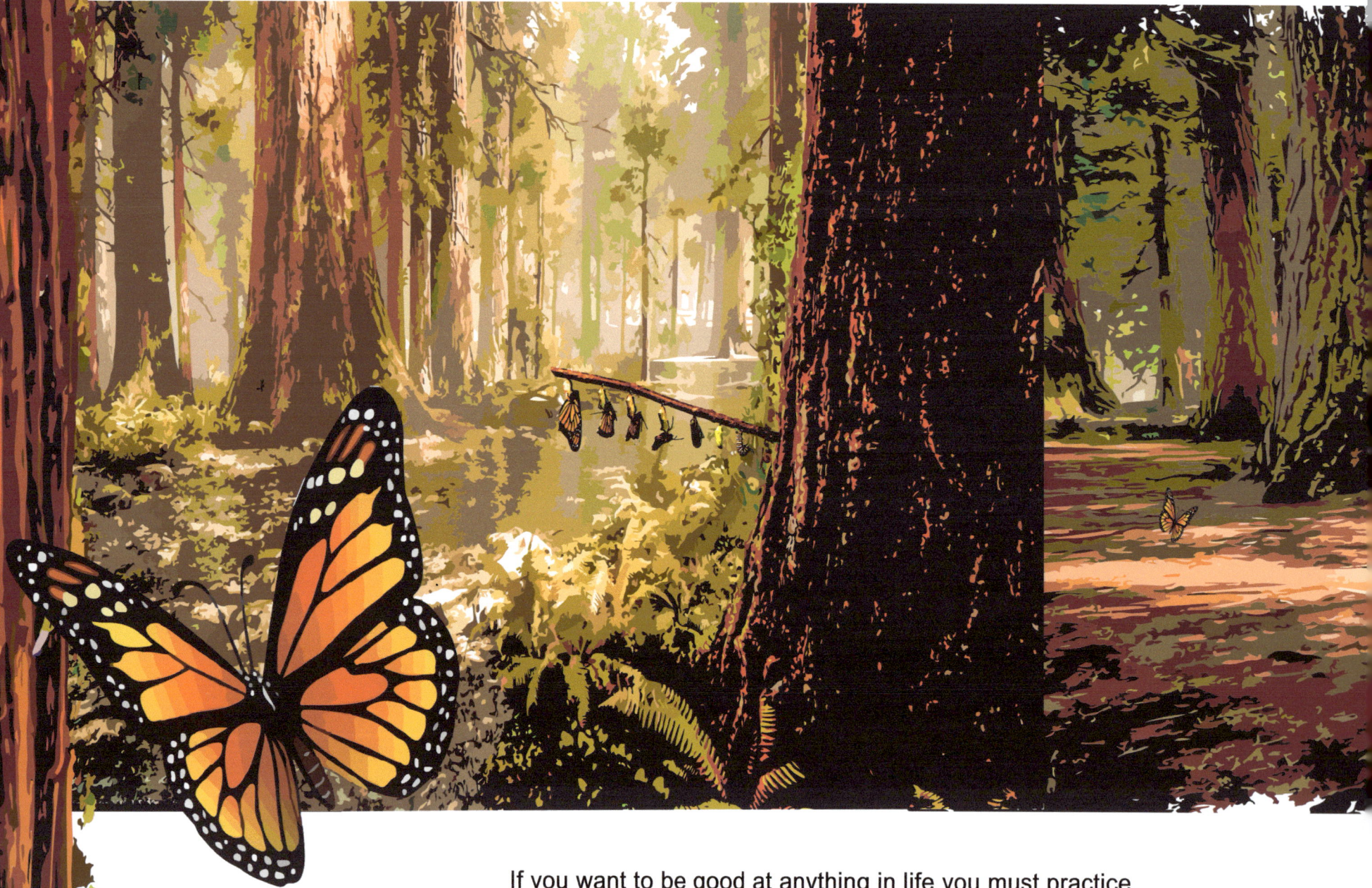

If you want to be good at anything in life you must practice.
Regular practice is the key; without it you will not progress.

I like to think of yoga as body mechanics; the how and why our body works the way it does. In a nutshell the body has three main parts to it: mind, body and spirit. The body is all the muscles, bones, joints, fluids and internal organs. The mind is the control room that oversees the functions of the body and the spirit is the motivating force that drives the mind.

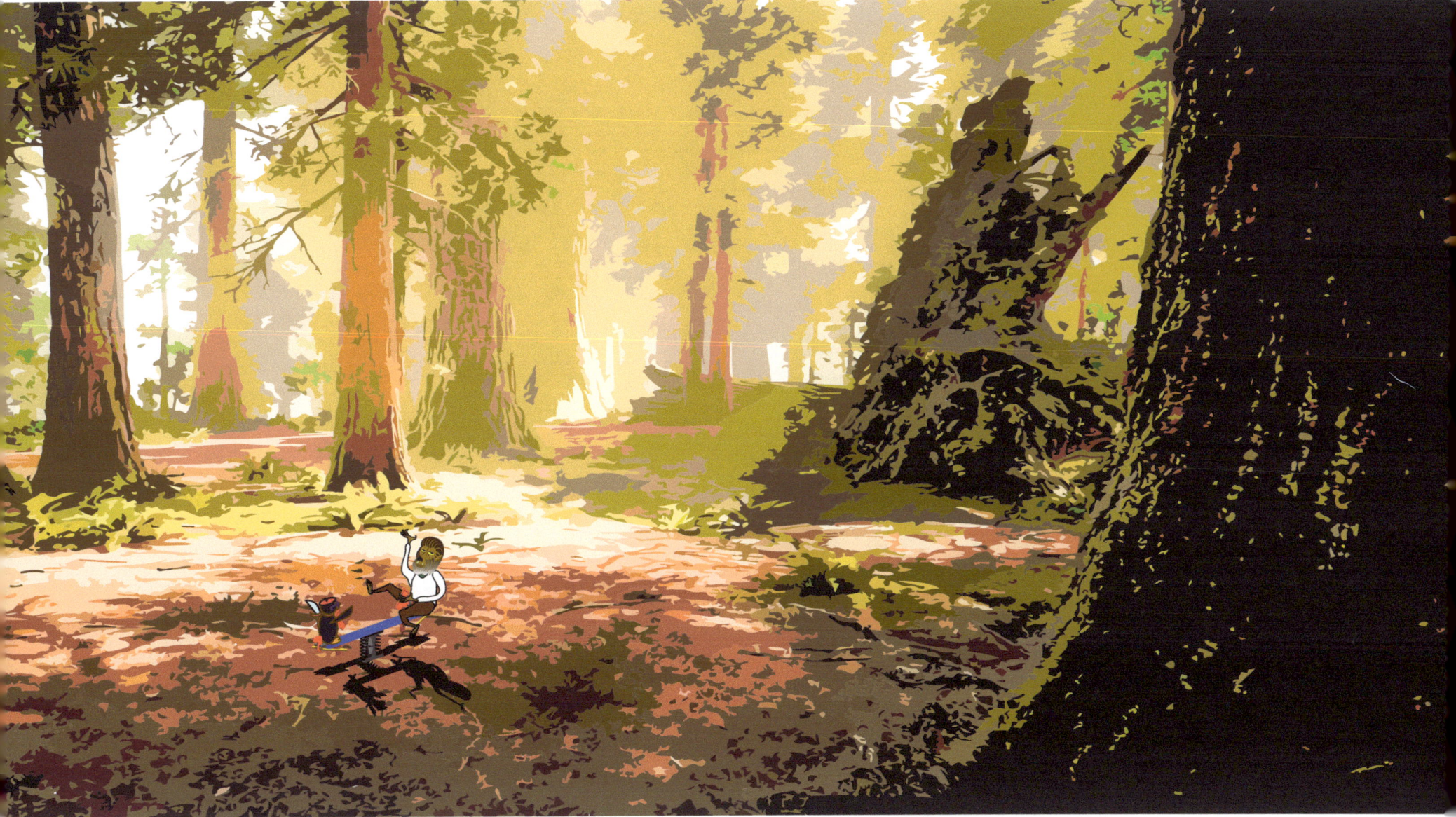

The Indian word yoga means union. If we cultivate a union or balance between mind and body, then we'll harmonise the spirit.
A wise person once said that the key to life is balance.

When you are born you receive two great gifts. The first is the earth and the second is your body. The Earth is where we live and the body allows us to experience it. This process is called life. Sometimes life can be quite difficult. We spend most of the time trying to avoid pain; physical pain, mental pain and spiritual pain. If we could feel no pain then life would be very easy.

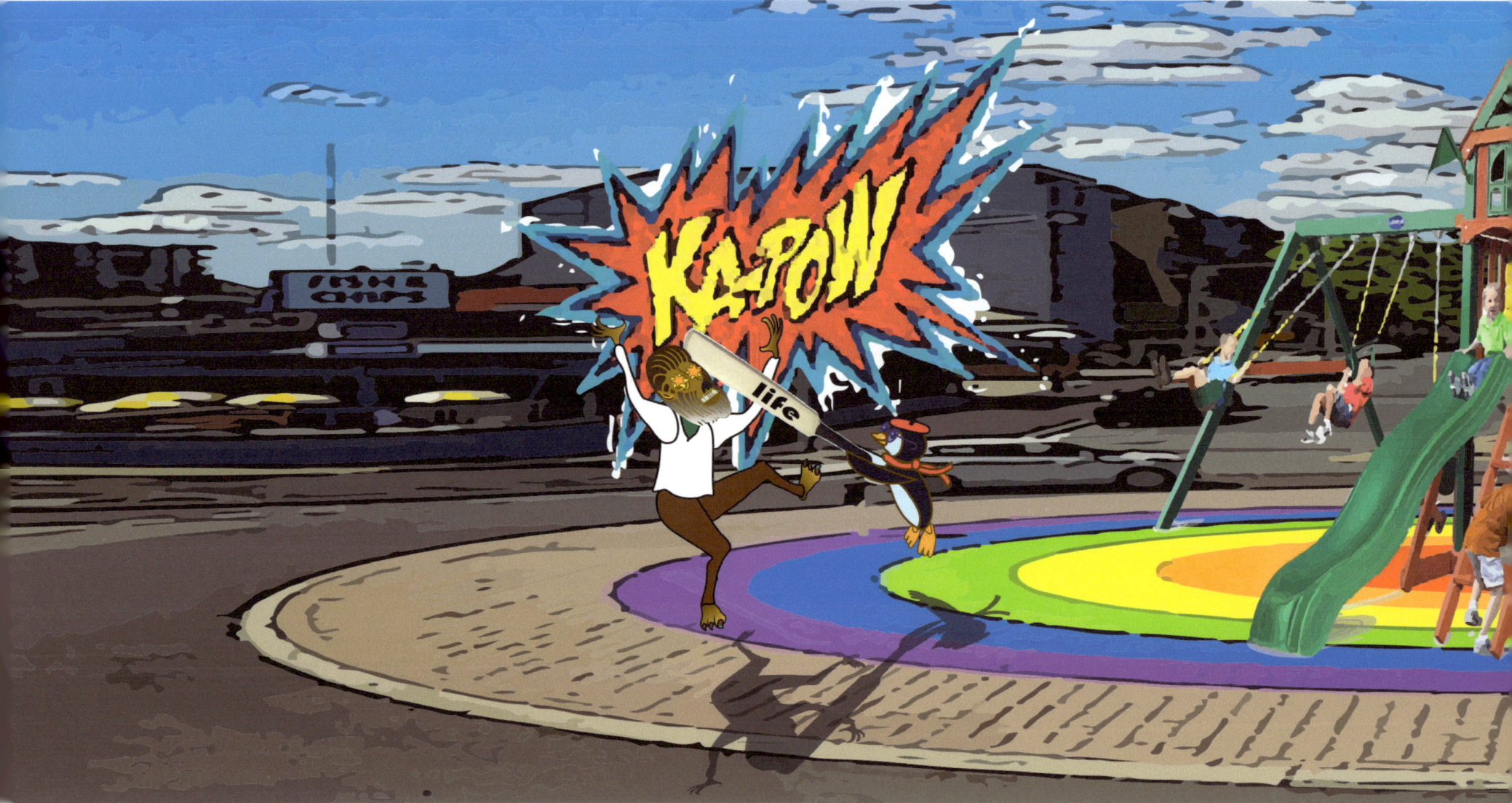

Most of us just want to be happy but life has a way of challenging us, which most of the time is heaps of fun, but can often be painful.

If you are born with a healthy body – ten fingers, ten toes, eyes, ears, nose, mouth and internal organs that all work properly then you are very blessed indeed. Sometimes people are born with parts of their body that are missing or that don't work properly. The awesome thing is that the body is so strong and adaptable that it learns how to function anyway. This is also a blessing.

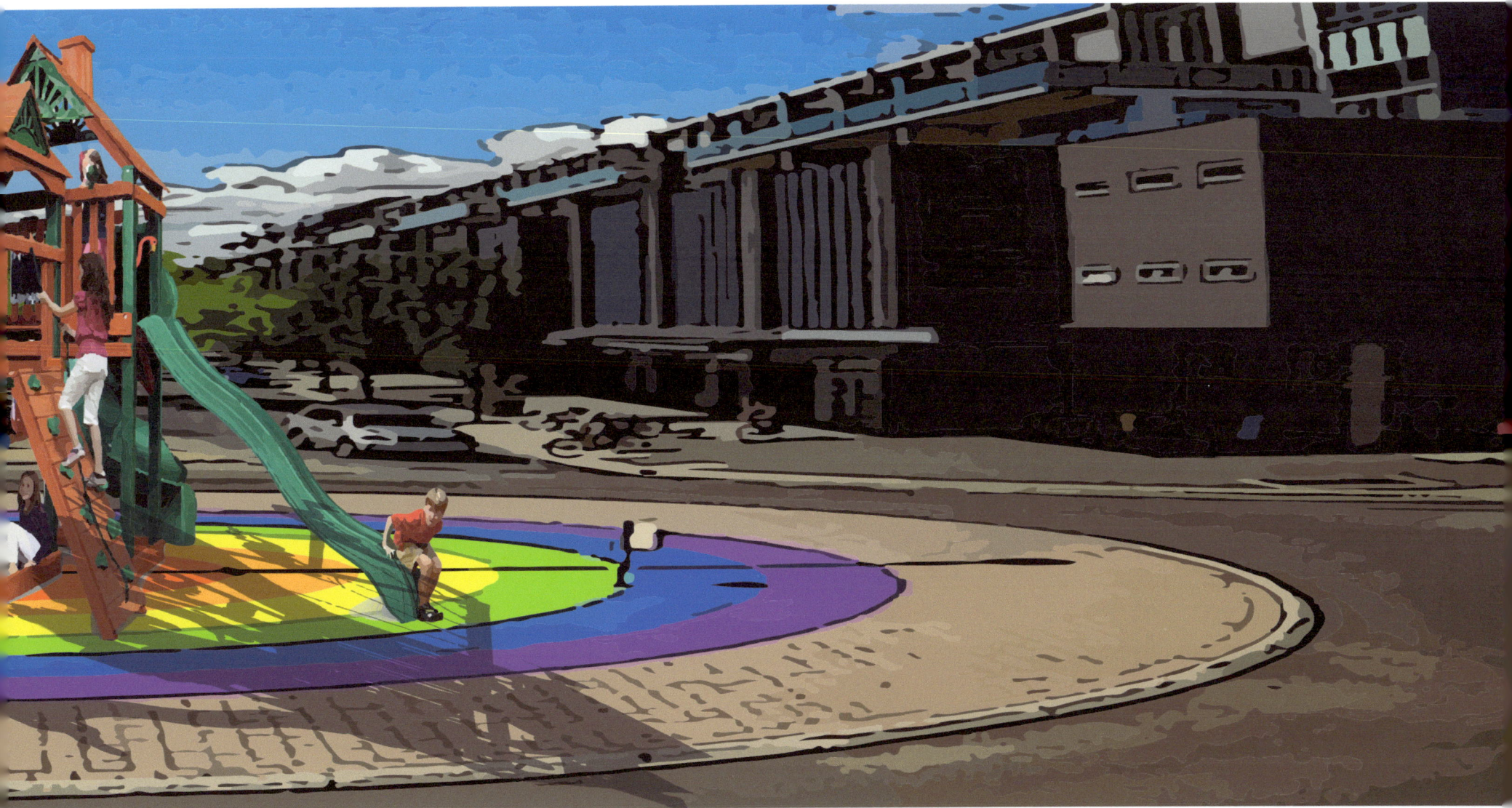

The tricky part is you have to live your life inside your own skin; you can't do it any other way.
You can't live outside of your body!
Living with yourself and others is one of the most challenging things you will do in life.

When you go to school they teach you how to live and work with other humans; this is called society or community. The problem is they don't teach you how to live with 'the self'; your thoughts, your emotions and your bodily functions, all the important stuff that happens to you on a personal level every day.

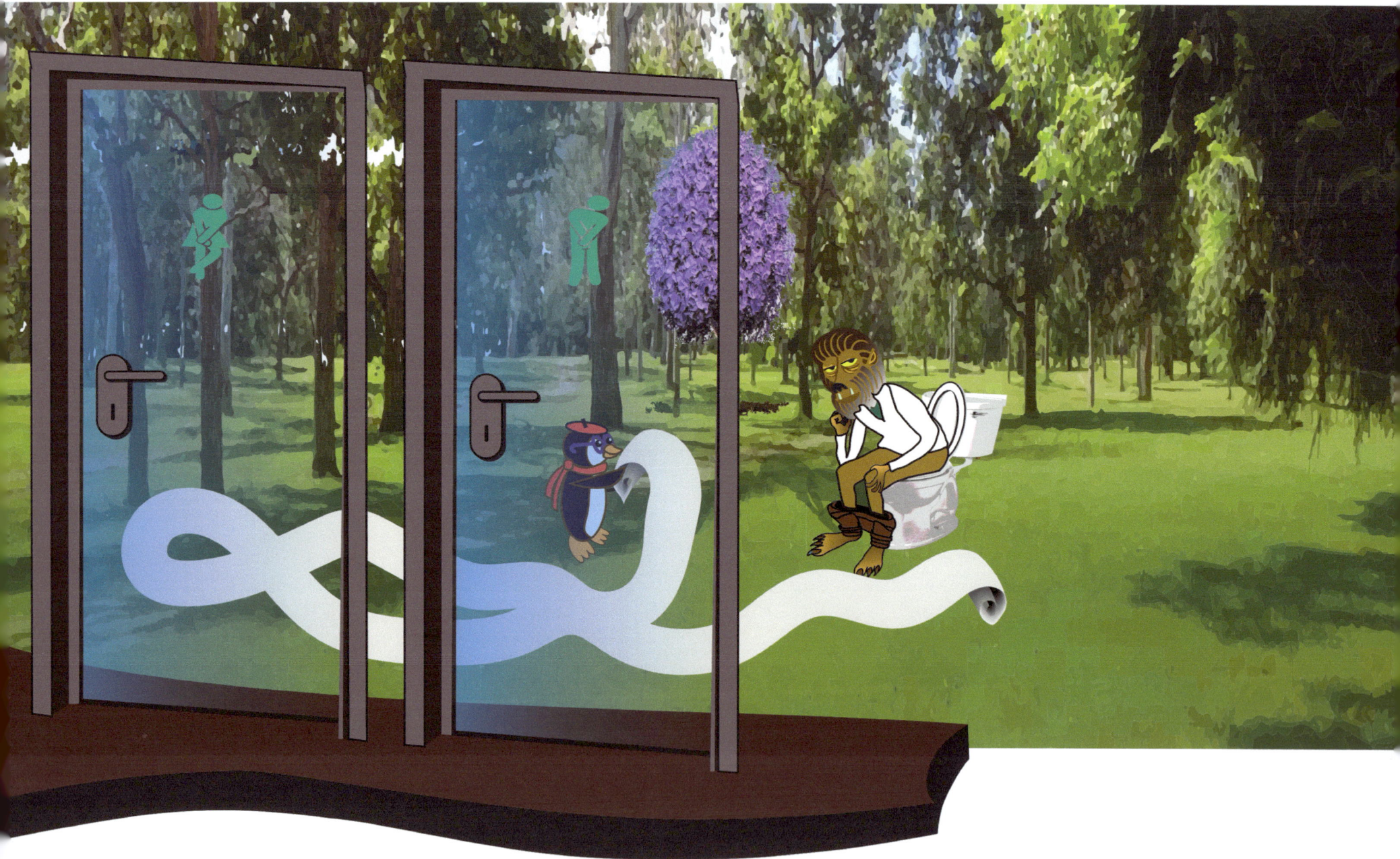

It's your parents' job to help you to understand all this stuff. They give you the basic training but most of the time they are too busy with their own lives to help you.

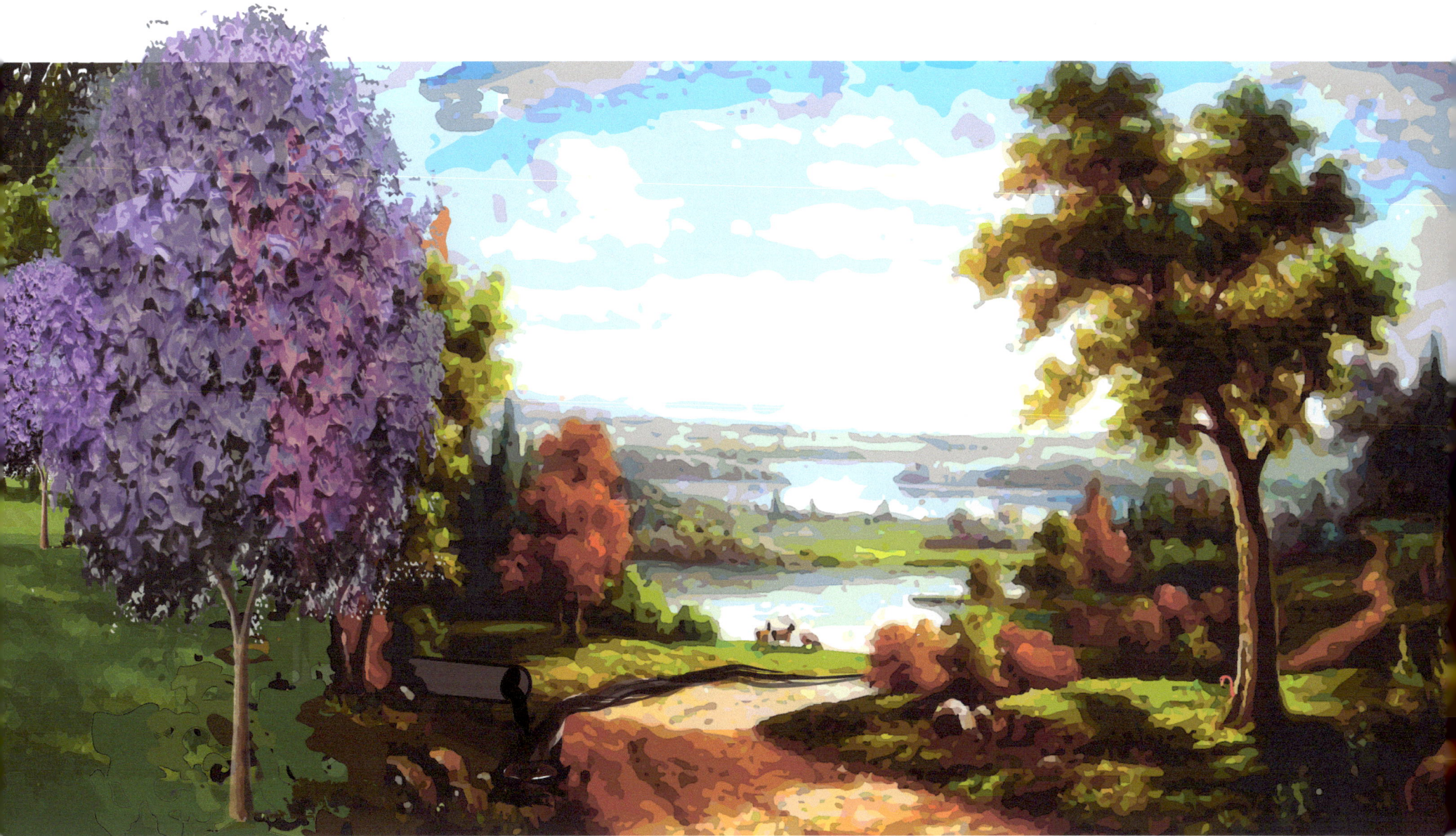

So the responsibility to understand yourself is up to you. It would be nice if we had some skills or tools to help us navigate and overcome problems that arise in the body. This is where yoga can help us. If yoga is the truth of the human body, then by understanding the truth we can understand how to be happy living inside of our own skin.

When we begin to study the body we see that it is a very complex system. The masters broke it down into five sections so it would be easier to understand; proper diet, proper exercise, proper thinking, proper breathing and proper relaxation. Each of these is a science unto itself

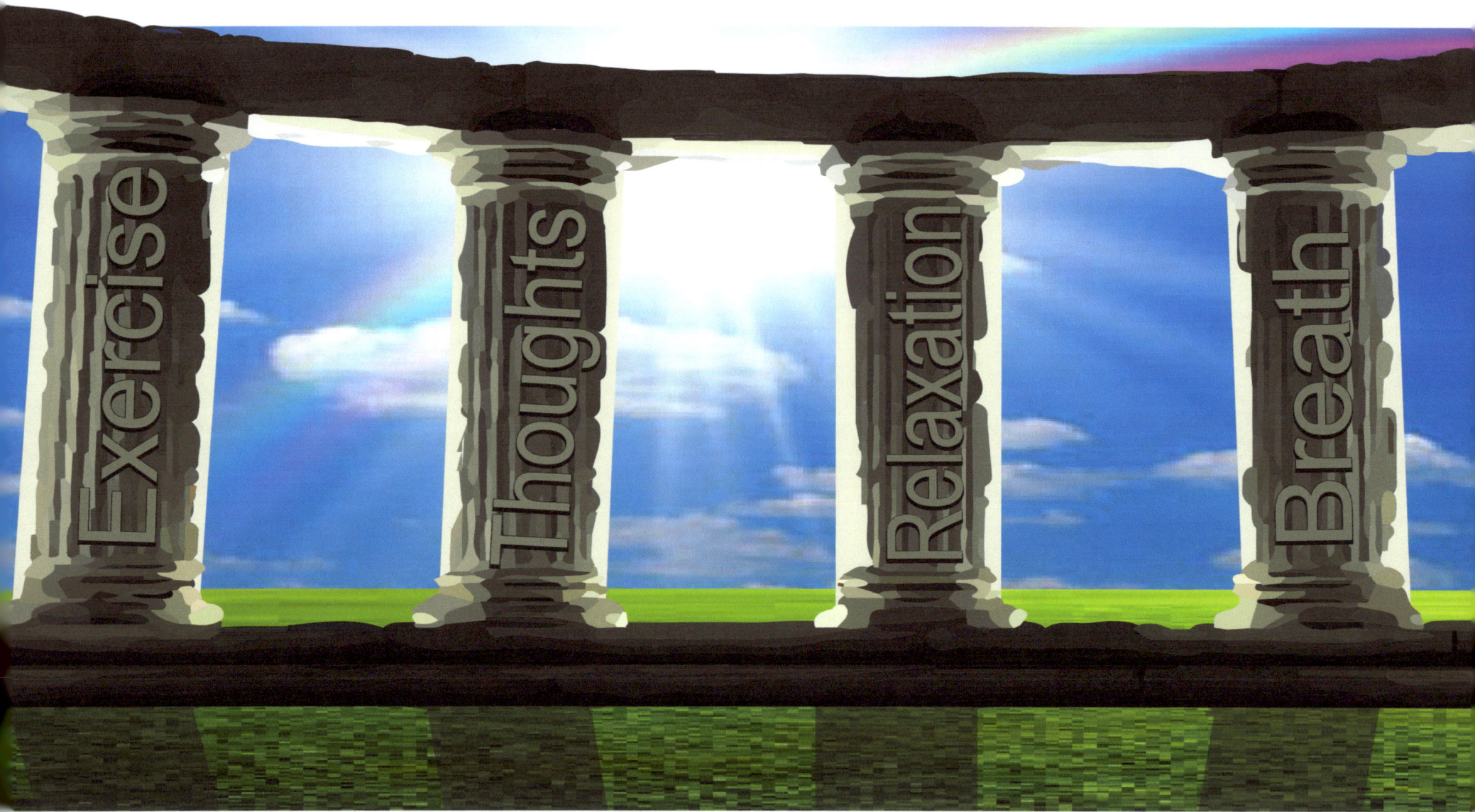

If we consider diet and how we fuel our bodies we learn that there are many different foods we can consume. Some are beneficial for the body and some are not. It's the same with thoughts. There are many good things we can think about and there are many thoughts that can cause harm. If we consider all thedifferent ways we can move our body, again some will cause pleasure and happiness and others will cause pain and its pain that we so desperately try to avoid.

If you have a bad diet, don't exercise, think bad thoughts, don't breathe properly and don't take time to relax, you will invite sickness into your life and make it very difficult to be happy. A good trick to life is; don't make it too hard for yourself. Life is already very challenging, you don't have to make it more so.

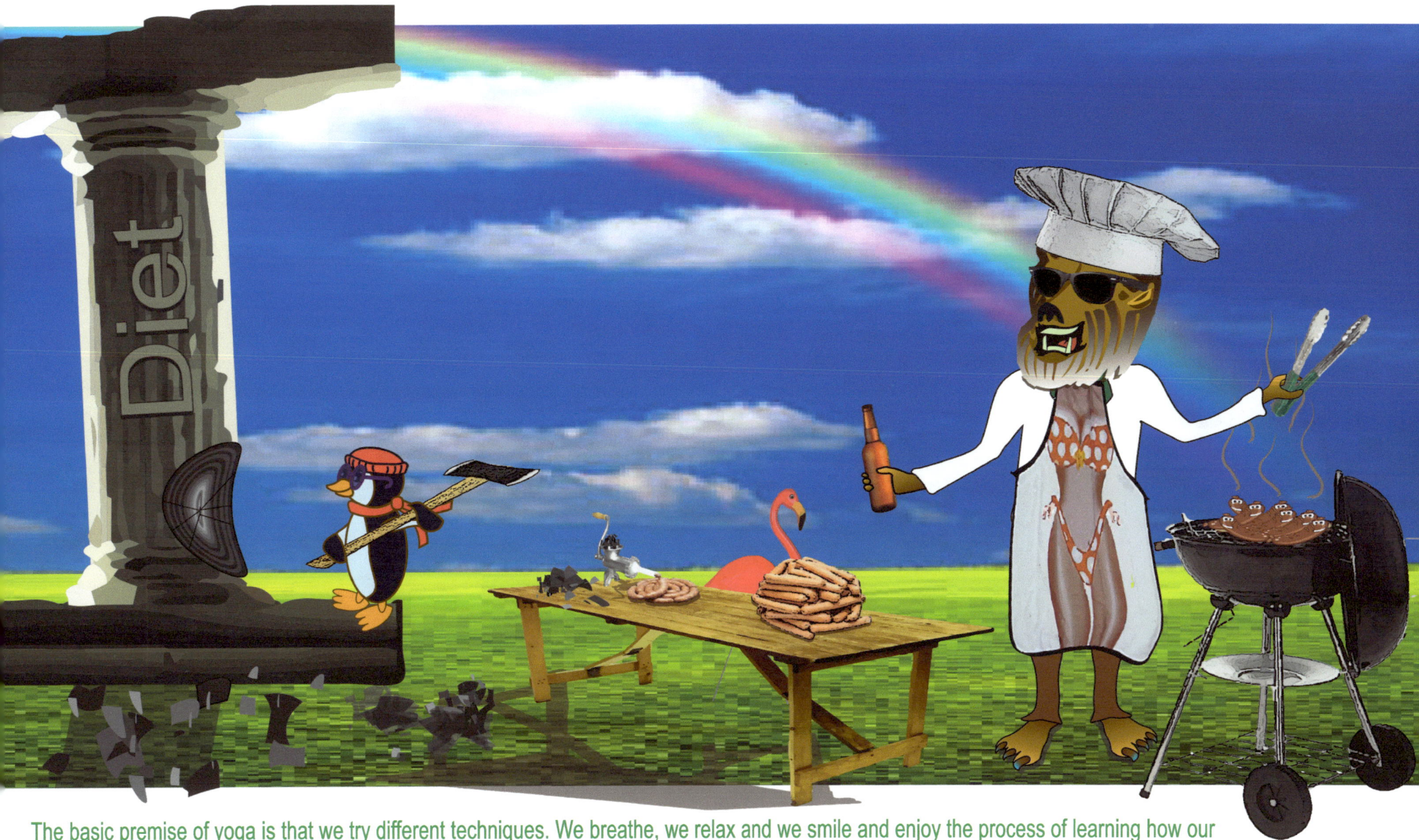

The basic premise of yoga is that we try different techniques. We breathe, we relax and we smile and enjoy the process of learning how our body responds. The body is your friend. You have to live with it every day. We like to help our friends and if we learn to understand our friends better, then we can enjoy a greater friendship. If your body is happy, you will be happy. If your body is sad, angry and in pain, you will feel the same.

Yoga is a very big subject. To give you an idea, there are more than 80,000 different ways you can move your body. In yoga these movements are called asanas. An asana is a steady, comfortable posture. Swami Satchidananda says; "if we can achieve one pose, that is enough. It may sound very easy, but in how many poses are we really comfortable and steady?"

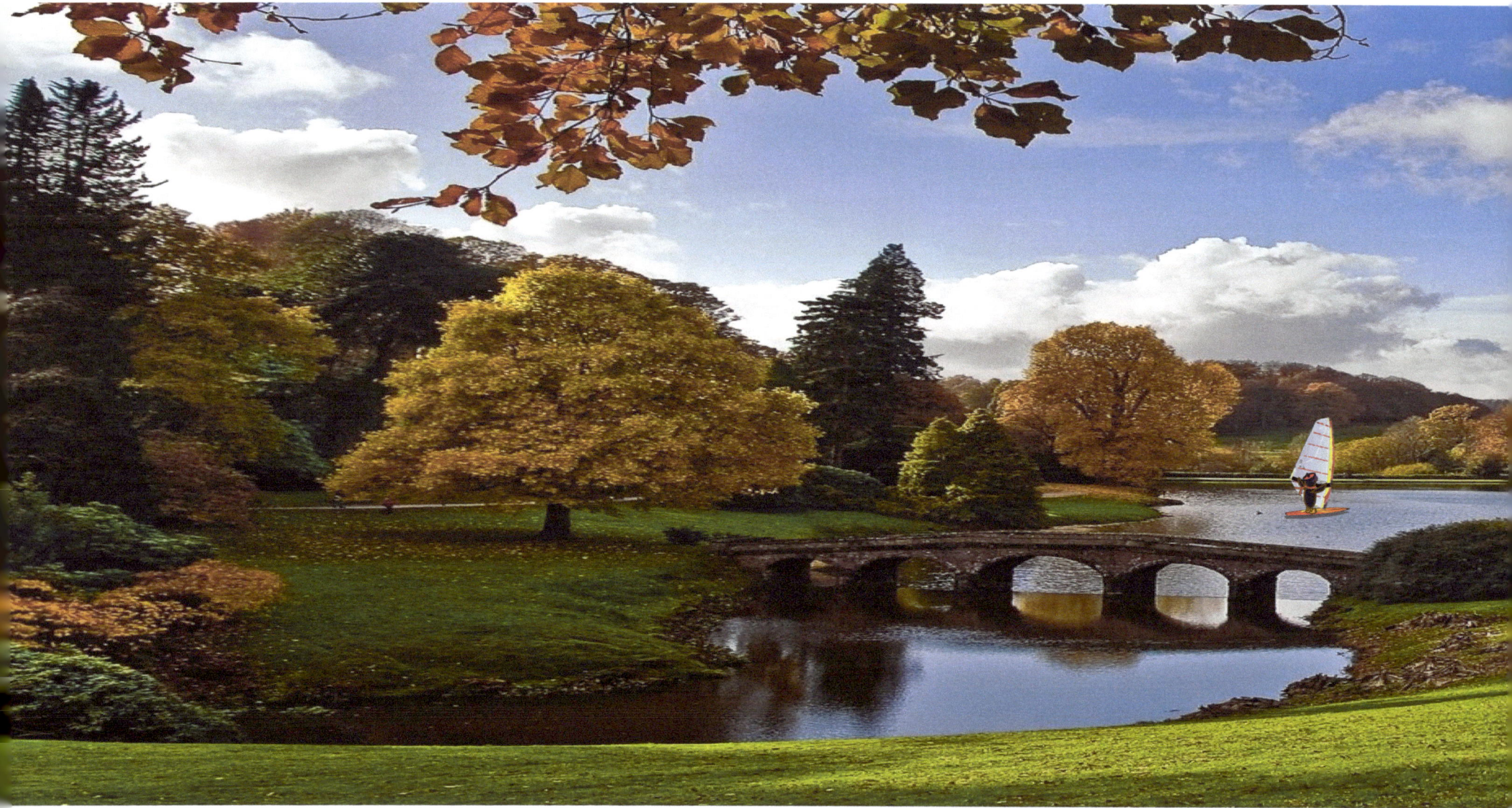

What we have to keep in mind is that not everybody is a swami (guru) or even a yogi (person who practices yoga), it takes many years to achieve this state of being. Some people may not even be interested in this lifestyle. However, yoga is for everybody, irrespective of race, culture, age, gender, religion or ability and by practicing a little and learning some skills, you can discover amazing benefits for yourself in a short time.

The beauty of yoga is that you don't have to do it all at once. You have the rest of your life to explore the subject. If you try a little from each of the pillars you will discover vast improvements and freedoms you didn't realise existed.

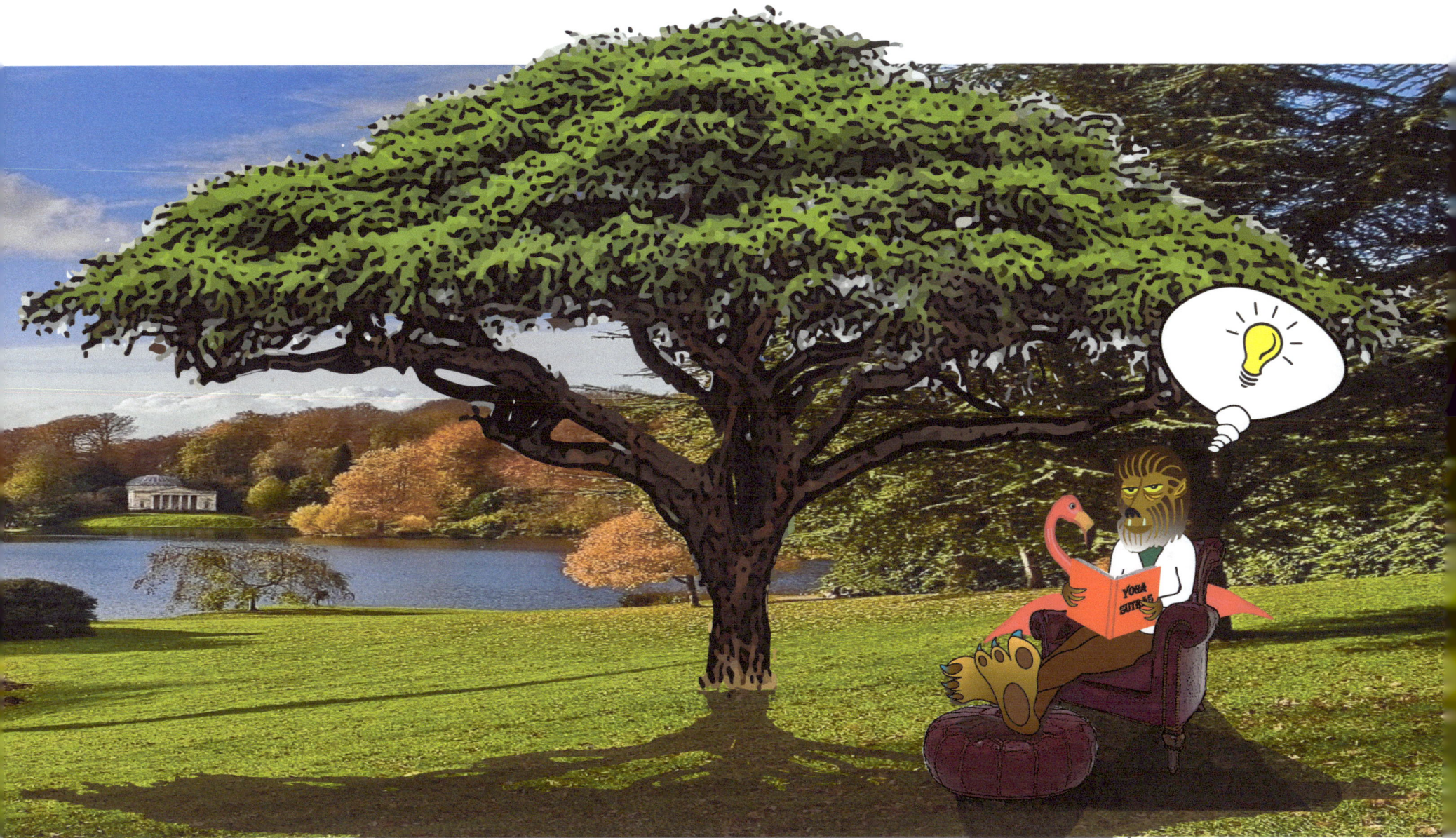

Amazing things will begin to happen. You will feel happier, more relaxed, more positive, less angry and anxious, health problems will disappear, you will develop better relationships with others, you will become more humble and appreciative of your surroundings and most of all your friends will see the change in you. This will inspire them to smile and share in your wellbeing.

Yoga usually begins with moving the body. In India when you move your body and you breathe and are conscious of the process, it's called yoga. In China the same process is called Qigong. The foundational pillar we are concerned with here is proper exercise or asana. The difference between yoga and everyday movement or exercise is that we are conscious of the breath before, during and after the movement.

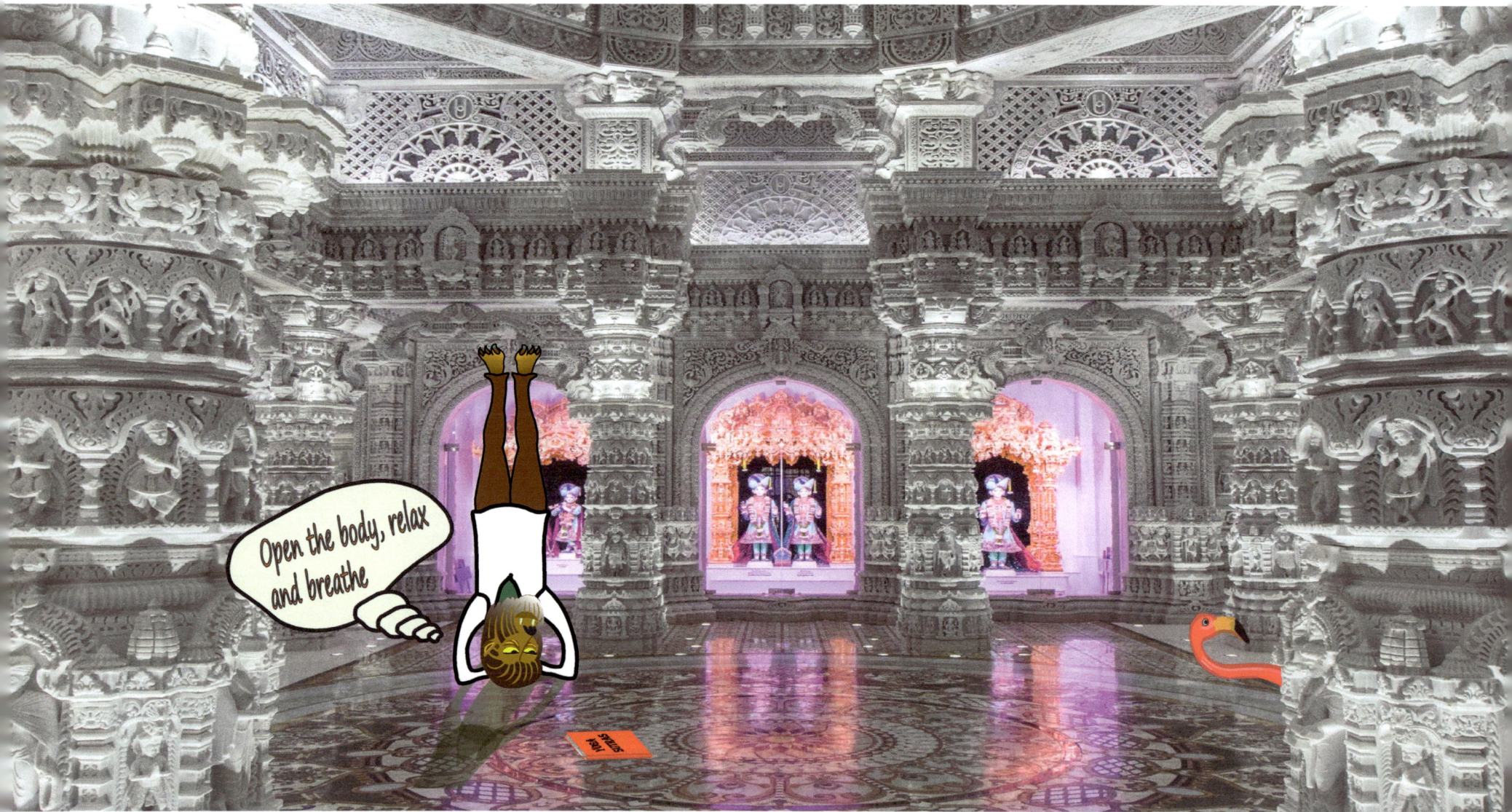

Open the body, relax and breathe

This awareness encourages us to think about three things; opening the body, relaxing the body and the quality of the breath. When we consider these three things during movement, we deepen and enhance the movement, yielding awesome results. The best part about yoga is that you already do it. It's a natural function of the human body. You relax the body when you sleep, you open the body when you yawn and stretch and you breathe when you inhale and exhale.

These functions are automatic; you don't have to think about them, they happen all by themselves. However, when you practice yoga, you do think about these processes which greatly enhances their effects on the body.

A wise person once said; energy flows where attention goes. This is what you capitalise on when you practice. You lead the mind to various parts of the body to energise, relax and rejuvenate muscles, bones and organs.

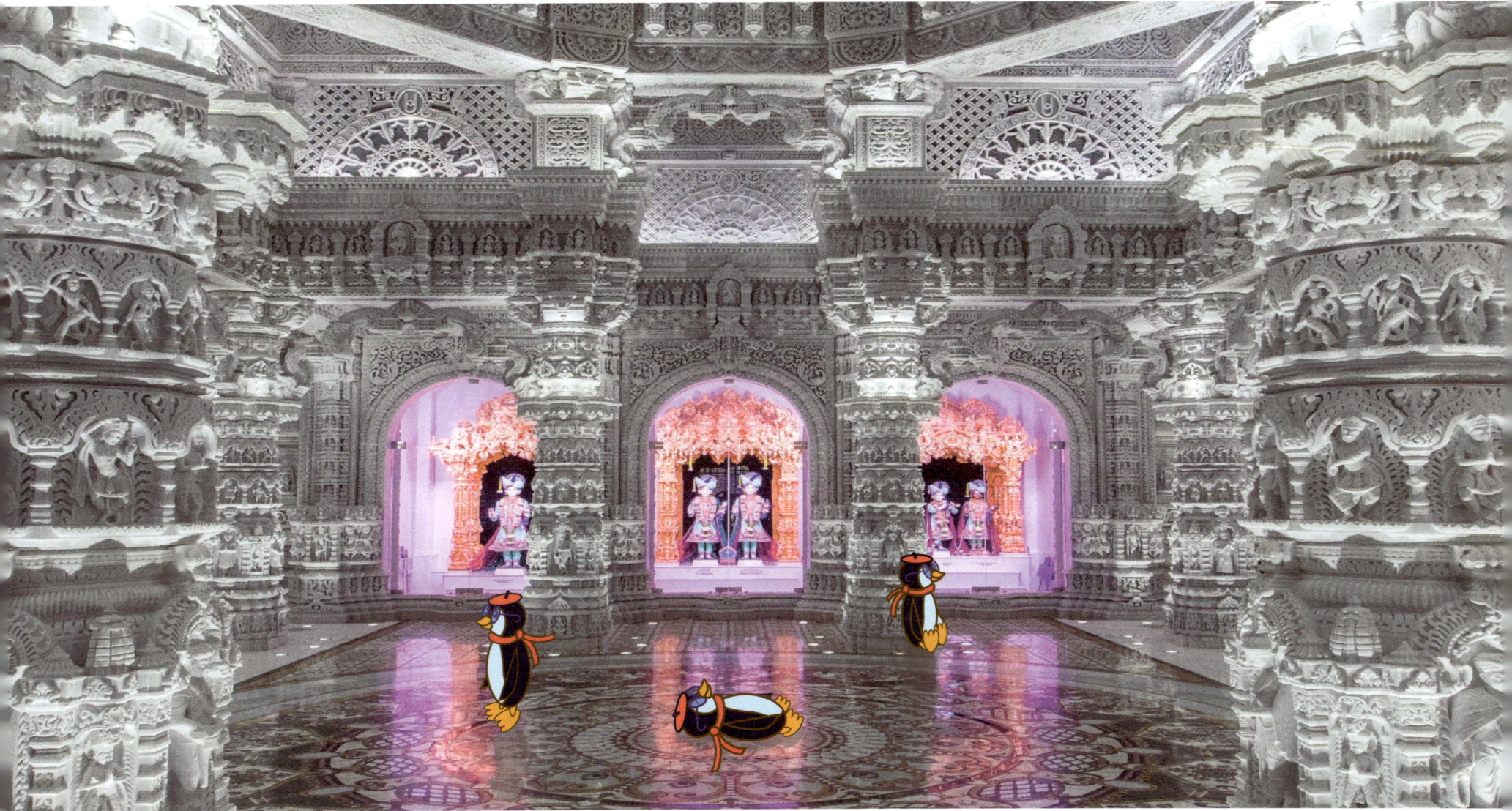

Sounds easy enough, but you have to focus and concentrate your mind on the task at hand which proves to be the challenge.

Of the 80,000 different asanas there are three main positions; Standing (Tadasana), Sitting (Sukhasana) and Lying (Savasana).

In each position we assume the posture, make the spine straight and focus the attention on the breath.

Tadasana – The Mountain Pose

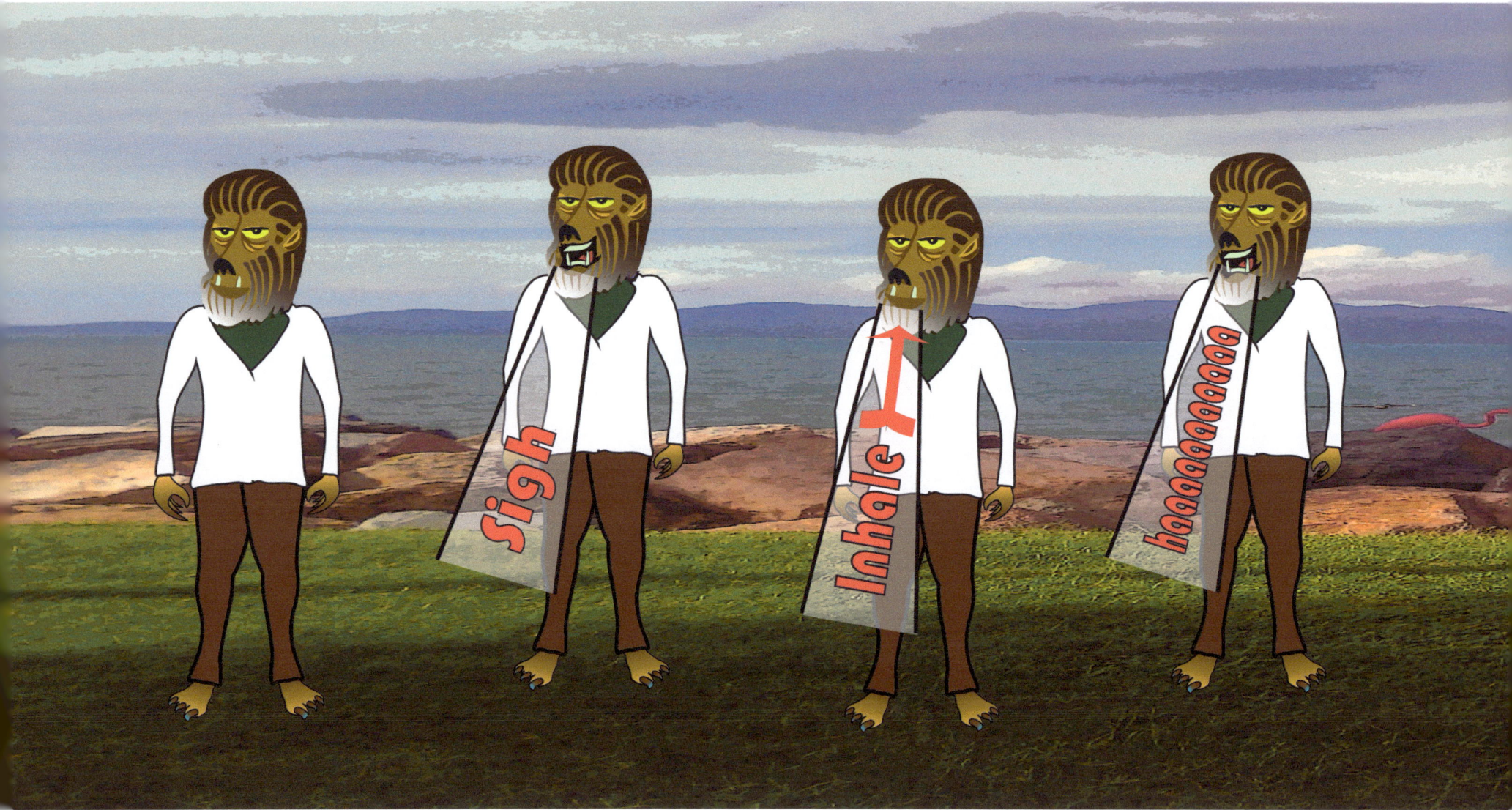

Begin by standing up straight, the feet are about shoulder width apart, arms hang by the sides and the body weight is evenly balanced. You need to relax the body so try some breathing. Take a deep breath and as you exhale enjoy a long sigh. Whisper the sound 'haaaaaaaaaaaaa' for as long as the exhale takes. Awesome. Now let's try it again. This time as you breathe out, making the sound, allow the body to relax as well. Repeat this process 10 times.

With each exhalation the body relaxes further. The muscles become soft and the mind becomes calm and quiet. Let go of any thoughts in your mind, you don't need them now, you can come back to them later.
Right now you focus on your breath.

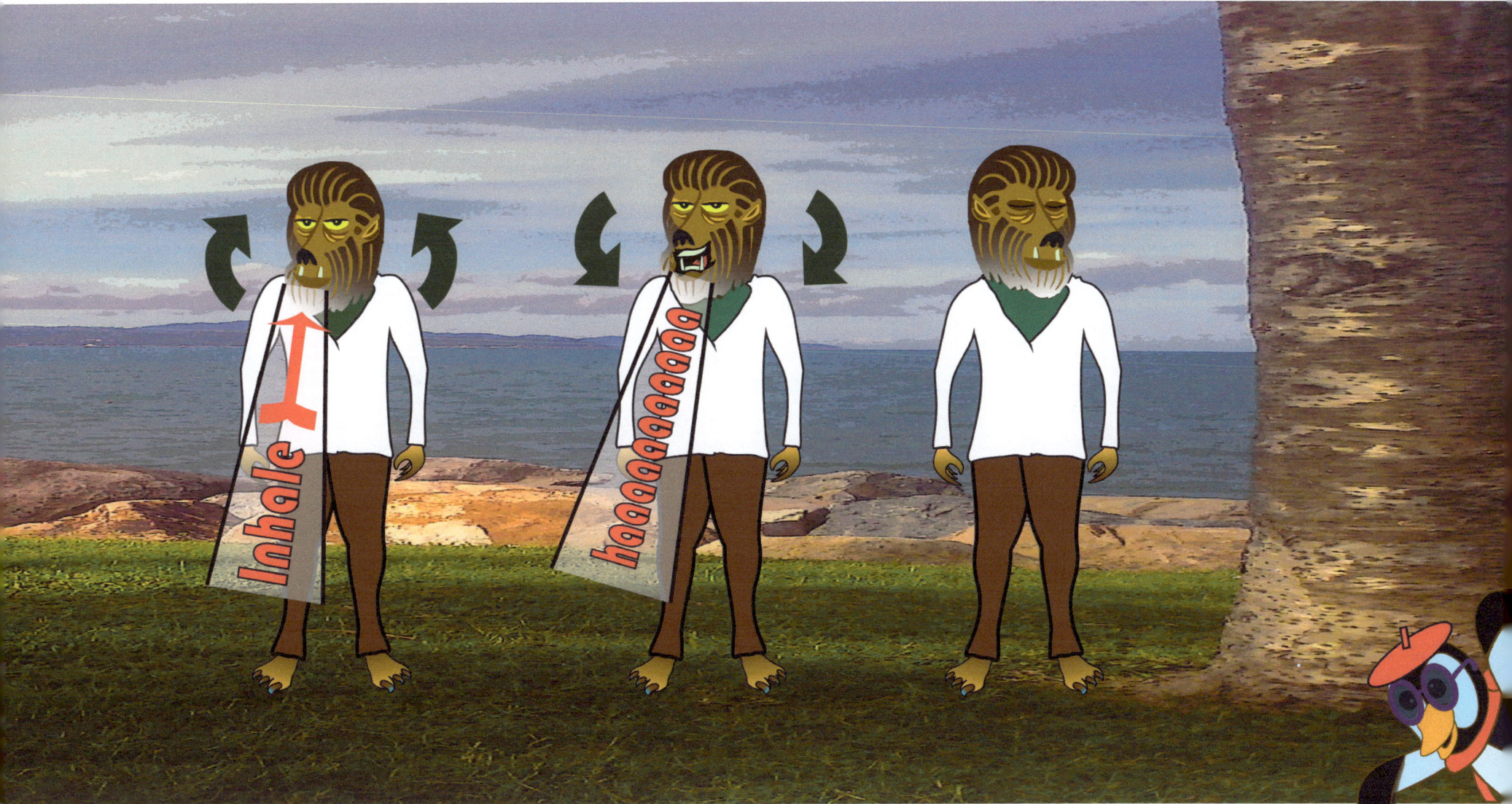

Let's add some shoulders. As you inhale lift the shoulders up. As you exhale let the shoulders relax down. With each exhalation the body relaxes further. Try it again. Enjoy the feelings of letting go and surrendering the muscles to the breath. When you finish, just stand quietly and notice how you feel.

Now without touching see if you can feel your spine. Move the head a little, feel the top of your spine. Move the pelvis a little, feel the bottom of your spine. Move your belly and ribs feeling the middle of your spine. By thinking of the spine it helps you to come into the present moment, known as 'here and now'.

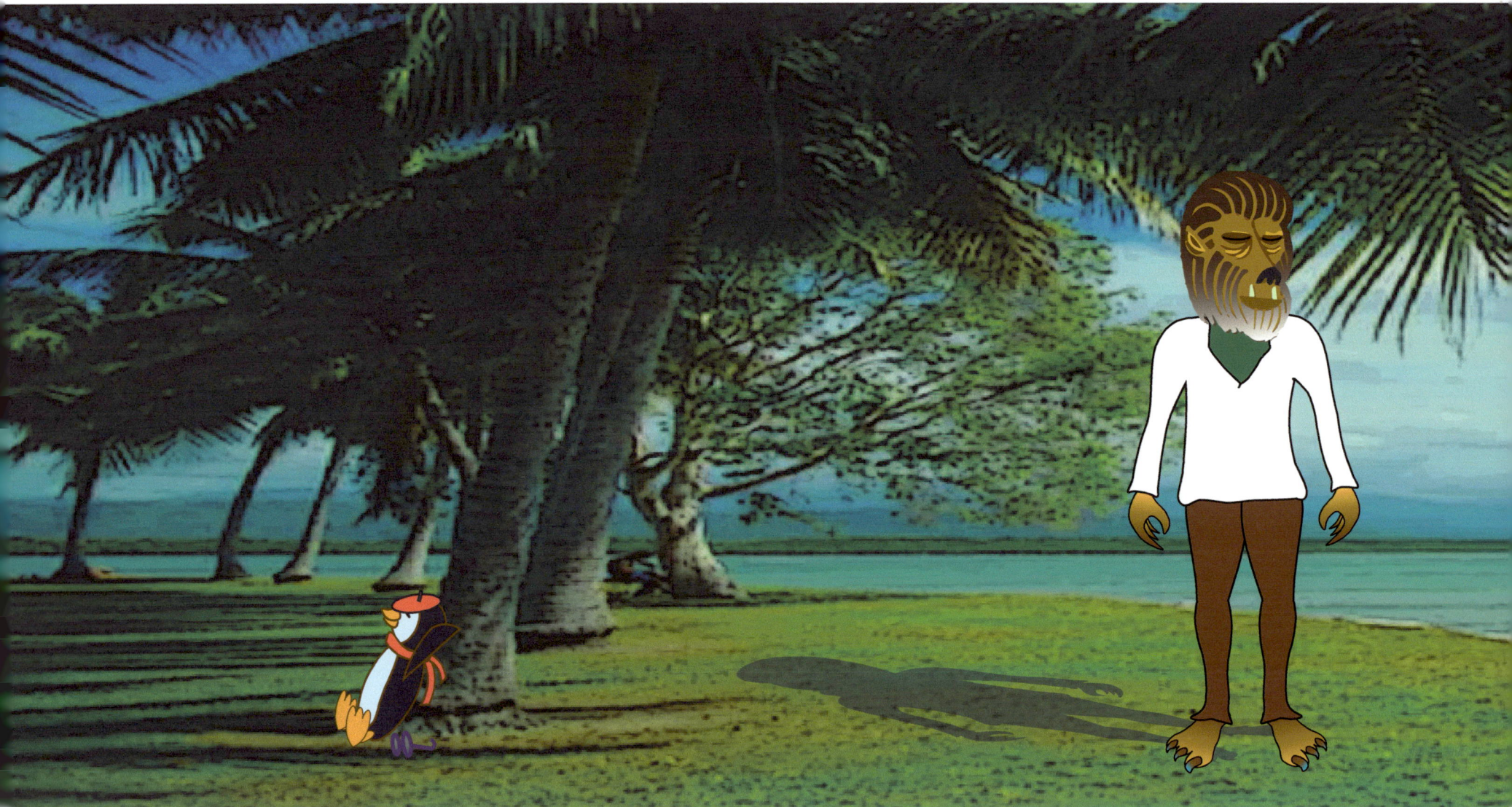

Think about making your spine straight; pelvis, hips, lower, middle and upper back, shoulders, neck and head all in a straight line. Tuck the tailbone under a little, maybe 1 cm and dip the chin down making the back of the neck straight. Soften the knees a little and let the arms hang limp by your side. Take a deep breath and relax. Beautiful, you're doing great, but you're only half way there. You still need to ground this posture and breathe into it.

Take your mind down to your feet and think about how your body weight is distributed. Shift the weight forward to the balls of the feet then back to the heels. As you slowly rock back and forth see if you can feel for the sweet spot in the middle where it's comfortable and easy to balance.

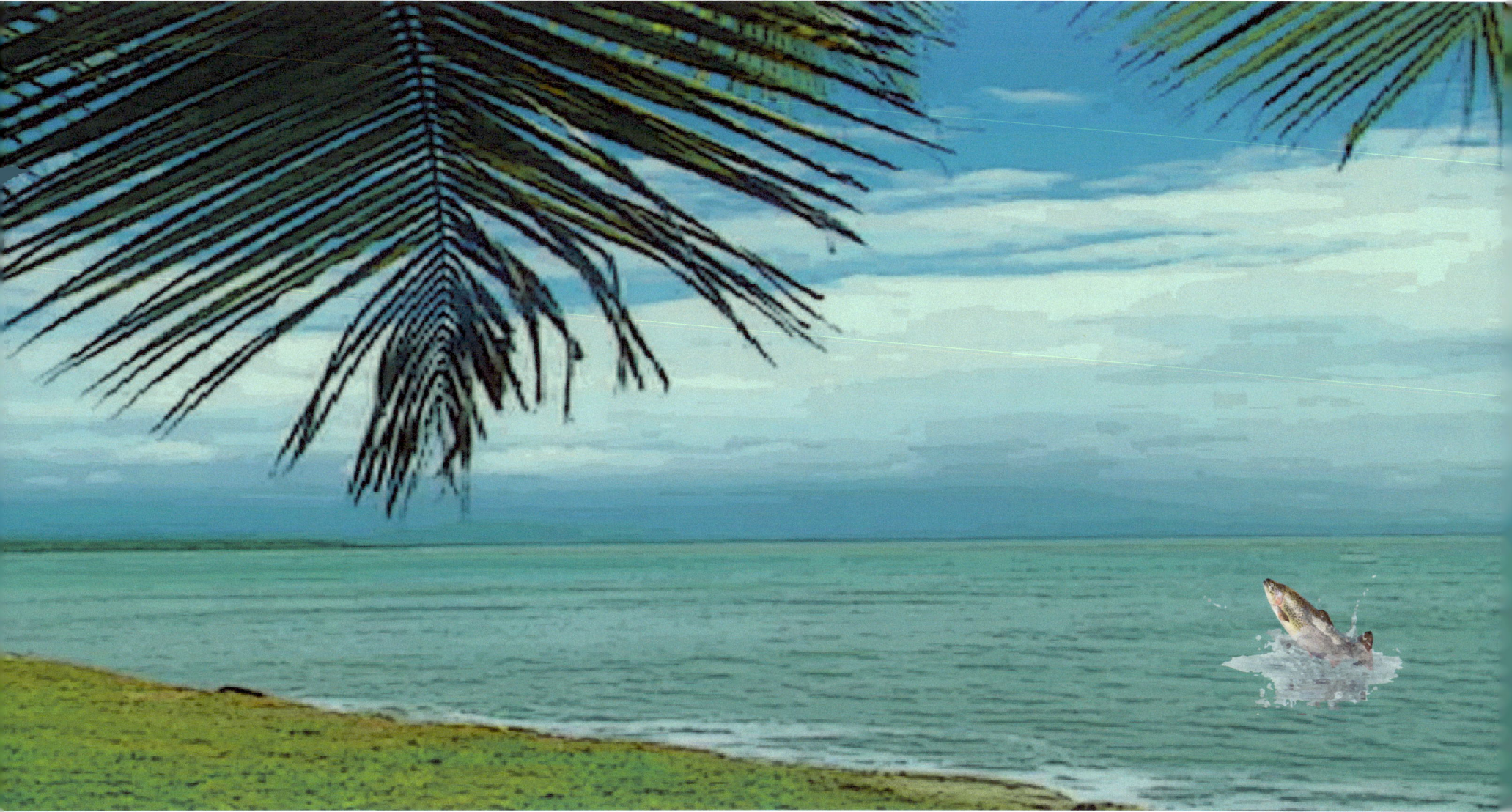

Now try rocking from side to side, left to right. Again feel for the sweet spot where your feet are nicely balanced. Spread out your toes and hold onto the ground with your feet. They should feel comfortable and centred. The body weight is evenly distributed. Take a deep breath. As you exhale think about your feet and the ground melting together. This exercise is called grounding. Take another breath and enjoy the connection to mother earth. It helps if you have bare feet and stand on the earth but it's not essential.

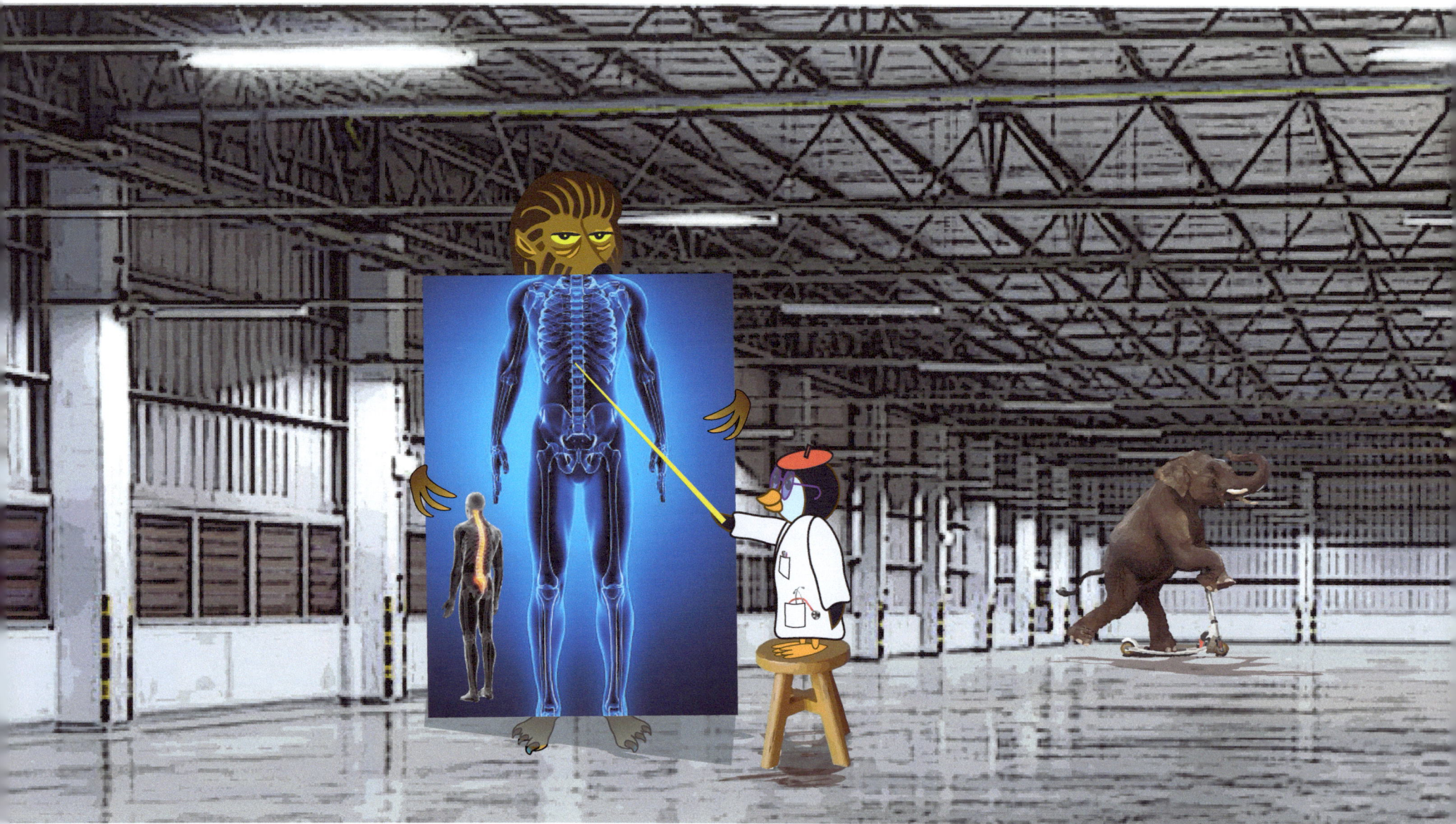

Once you establish this connection you want to stand up straight. Think about lifting up and opening your heart, take the shoulders back and imagine a piece of string connected to the top of your head that lifts your skull upwards. Remember to keep the chin dipped down a little and the arms relaxed by your side. Take a nice deep breath, as you exhale allow all the muscles in your body to soften and sink down. The skeleton stays up straight and erect but the muscles relax down.

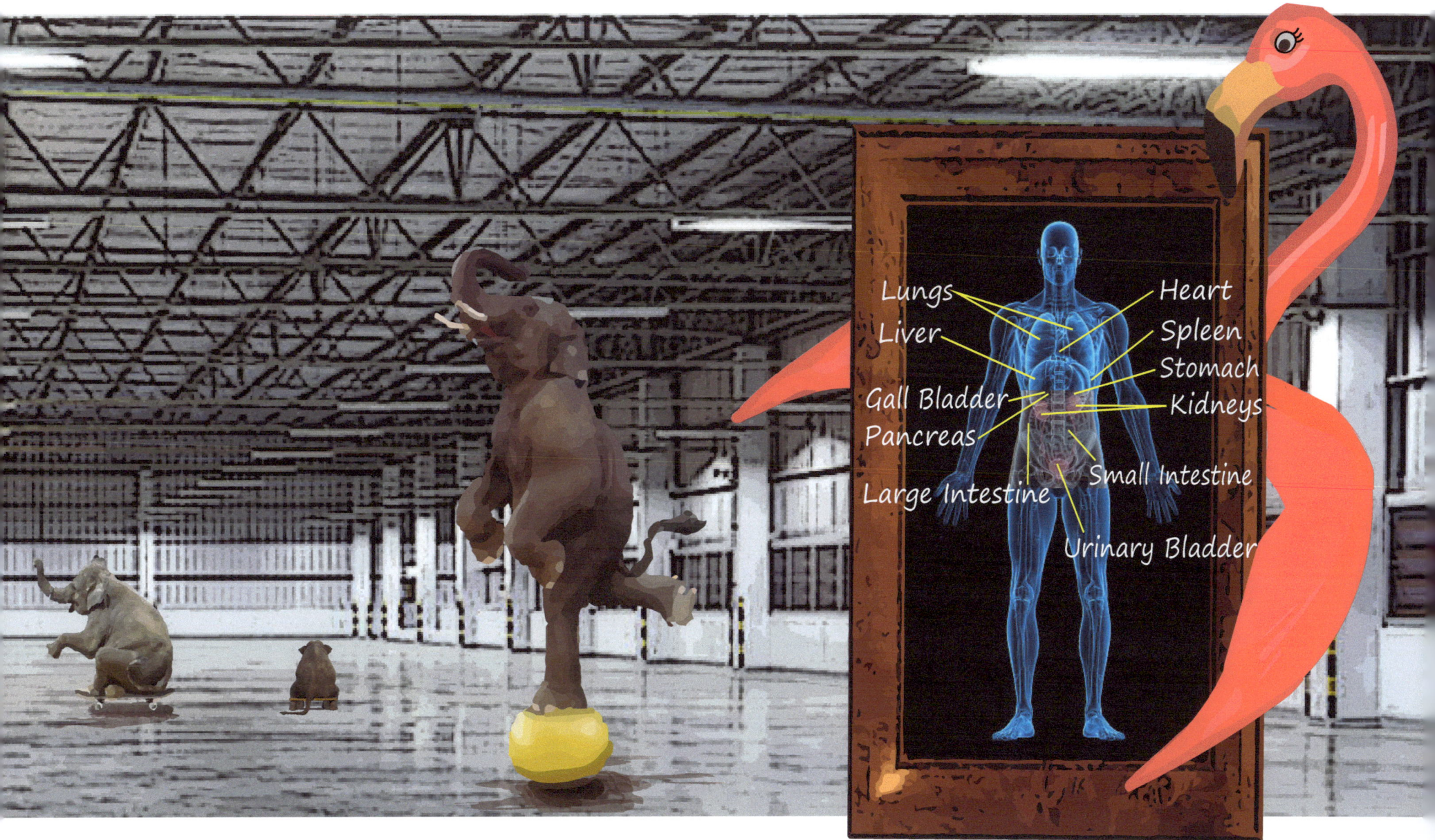

Lungs
Liver
Gall Bladder
Pancreas
Large Intestine

Heart
Spleen
Stomach
Kidneys
Small Intestine
Urinary Bladder

Take another breath. As you inhale allow the oxygen to expand in your lungs.

As you exhale smile to yourself and enjoy the relaxing feeling.

Try this for another 10 breaths. There's no rush, take your time and focus on what you're doing.

Think about standing up tall and proud like a mountain.

As you inhale think 'quiet'. As you exhale think 'relax'. You can close your eyes if you like. With each exhalation the whole body relaxes further, the muscles feel nice and soft, the mind is calm and quiet, the spine is straight but not strained and the breath is smooth and slender.

This is Tadasana, the mountain pose, the first standing posture. It's really cool!

Don't worry if you don't get it at first, there are a lot of things happening, it takes a bit of practice to co-ordinate everything and get it right. The cool part is that the more you practice the easier it becomes, you'll feel more confident and your mind will be calm, focused and quiet.

This my friend is yoga!

While you were busy thinking about breathing, grounding, straight spine, opening the heart, shoulders back and relaxing, you weren't thinking about friends, school, work, children, chocolate or how upset you were or anything else. The mind was completely in the moment focussed on the task at hand. You opened the body, relaxed the body and oxygenated the system.

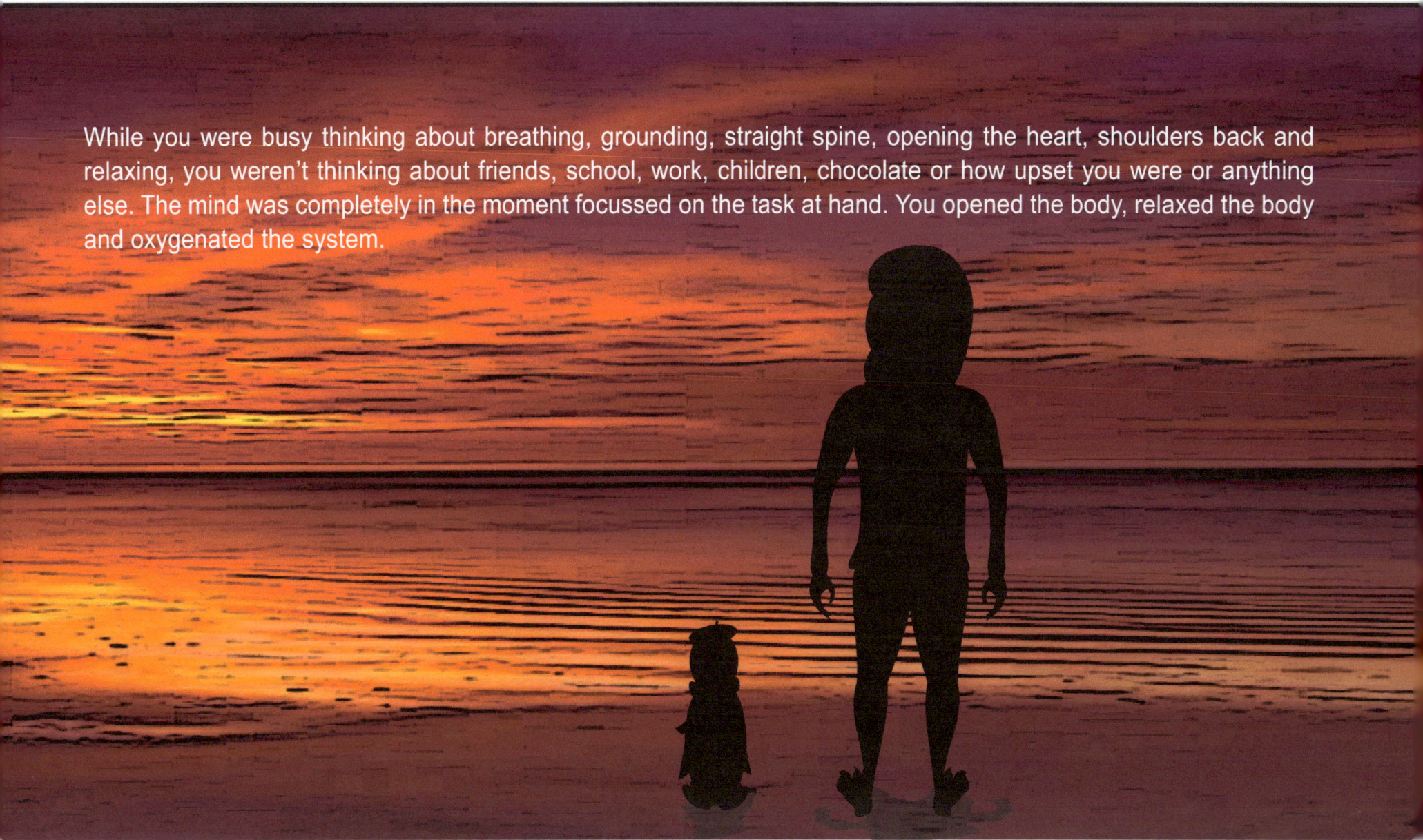

Congratulations!
If you can do this asana you can repeat the process for other asanas.

When you practice yoga there is one golden rule to keep in mind; if it doesn't feel right for your body, then don't do it. Stop and move onto something else – you don't want to hurt yourself.

Big Breaths

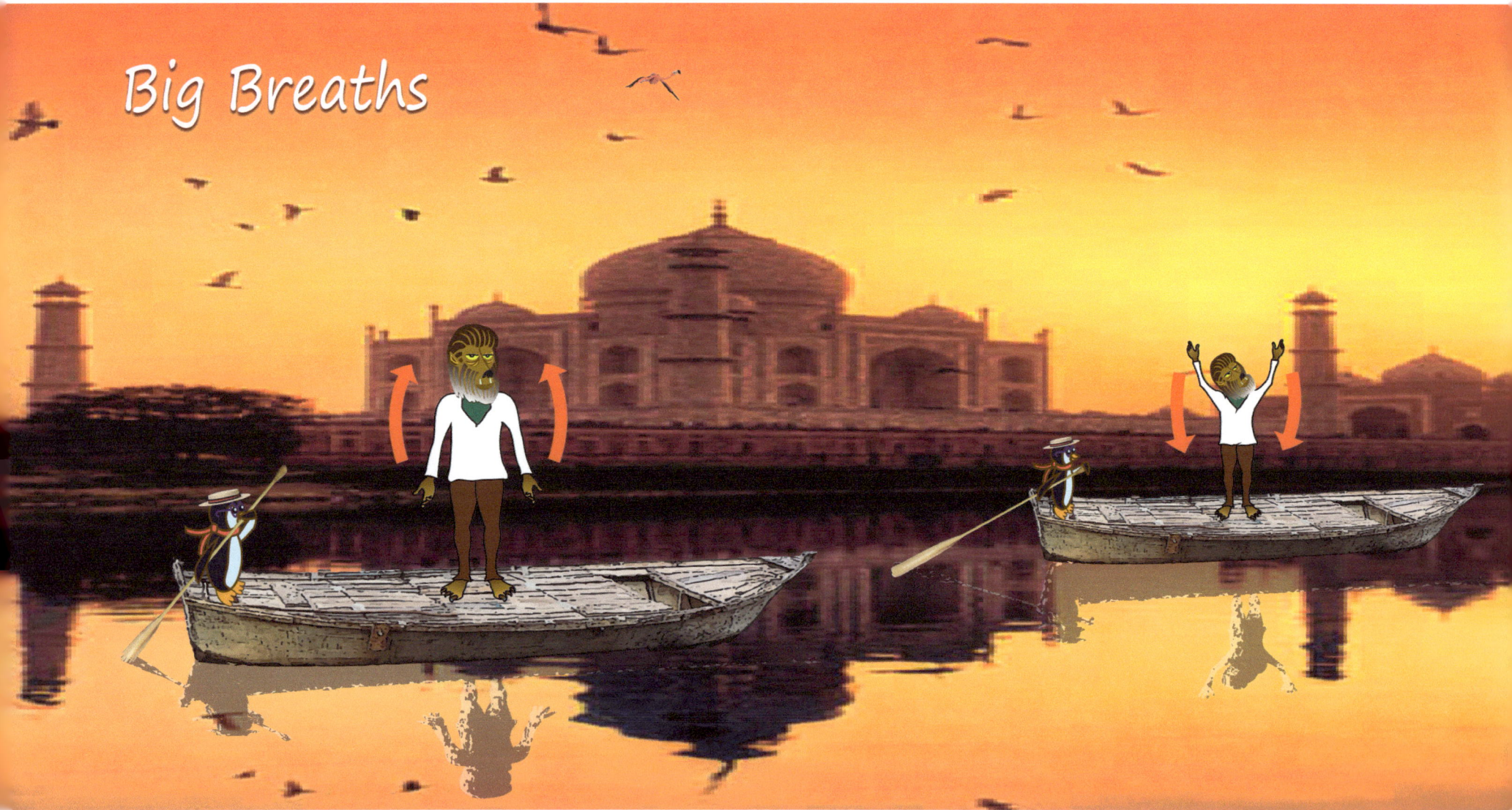

The idea is that you are trying to open your body, learn some new things and enjoy the process. Pain is not part of the equation. Yoga is very easy, it doesn't need to be difficult. At times it will be quite challenging, this is how you learn. When you try too hard or strain yourself you will hurt yourself. It's just like a fire; you want to be close enough to feel the warmth and goodness it provides but not too close that you burn yourself.

Yoga is very powerful. Just by putting your body in different positions you can enjoy amazing results. You don't have to try too hard. Just relax and have fun.

Let's begin to move and open the body. Start by opening your palms and floating the hands up above your head. Then turn your palms over and float your hands back down by your side.

Try again but with some breathing too. Inhale as you float your hands up, exhale as you float them down. Try to coordinate the movement with the breath, then slow it down to find the rhythm of your body.

Next try including the head.
Inhale, float the hands up, look up.
Exhale, float the hands down, look down.

Repeat this movement about 10 times

In your mind think about making the movement soft and slow. Long, deep breaths and a smooth, relaxed movement. Imagine you're a big bird flying high in the sky. Feel your way through the movement. Feel the muscles and the joints that are moving and breathe into them. There's no rush and there's no right or wrong. Just have fun.

Reach for the sky and touch the toes

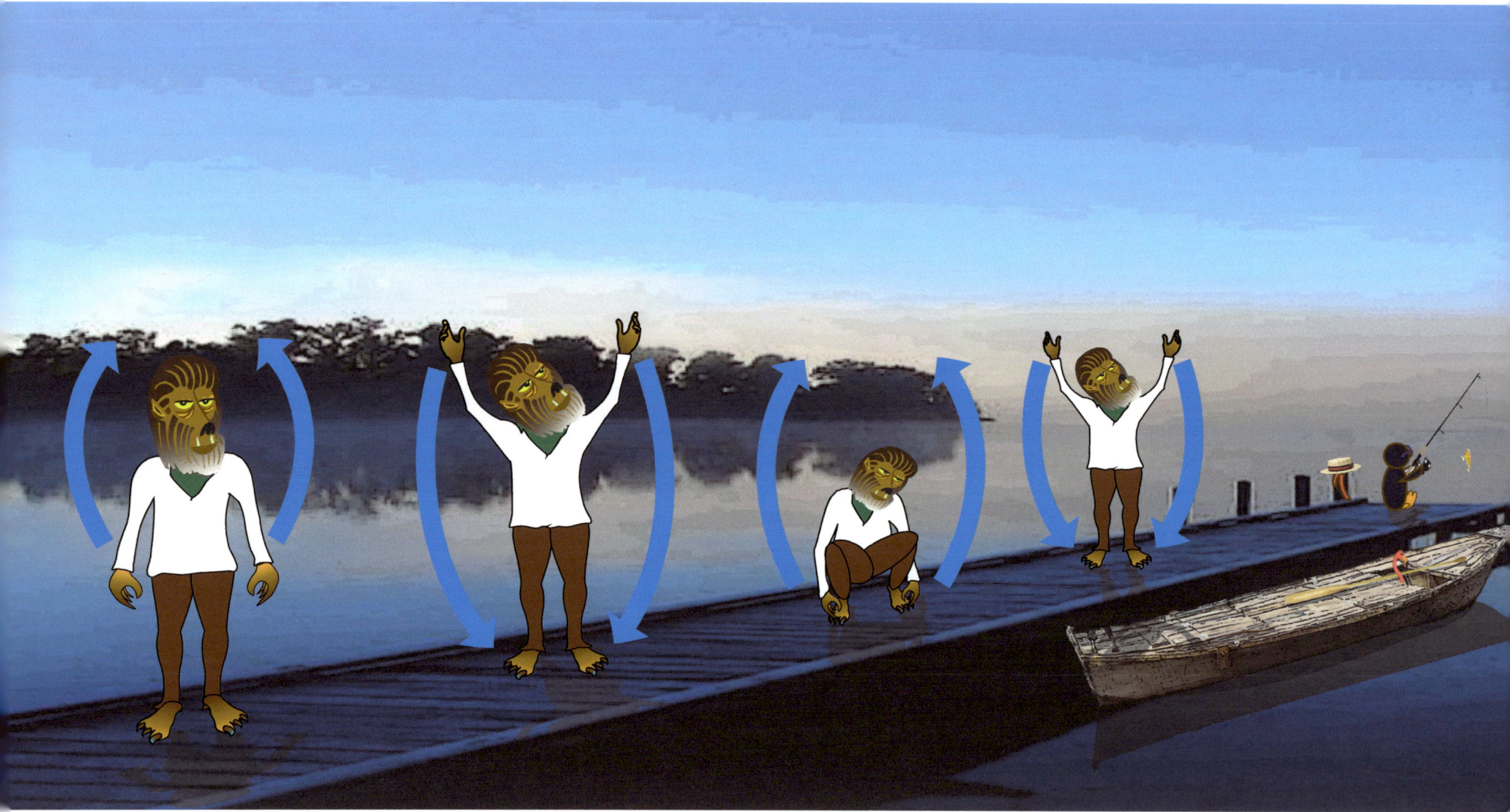

When you breathe you want to breathe through your nose. Breathe in the nose, breathe out the nose. If this doesn't work for you then just do something that's comfortable and does work. In yoga you are moving towards an ideal, it's a progression of learning and you get better the more you practice. So if you can only breathe through your mouth today that's a great start.

Extend this movement now to reaching down and touching your toes. First inhale and float your hands up to the sky. Then soften your knees, exhale and float down to touch your toes.

Inhale, rise up, look up.

Exhale, float down, look down.

Repeat this about 10 times. Each time think about taking long deep breaths and making a smooth slow movement. When you slow the movement, you slow the breath. When you slow the breath you slow the heart and when you slow the heart you relax.

Pretty simple isn't it?

This beautiful yet easy move is a great way to open the body and get the breath and body moving together. You could try ten in the morning when you wake up, it only takes a minute but gets your body feeling great and ready for the day.

It would be the same if you did ten before going to bed. The body is open and relaxed, the system is oxygenated and you can sleep better. In fact you could try this at any time of the day. Give it a go and find the best time for your body.

Start in the mountain pose, tadasana. Do you remember the mountain? Stand up nice and straight, make the spine straight, shoulders back and relax. This time step your feet out a little wider than shoulder width. Bend your knees to reach down and pick up an imaginary basketball off the ground. Now lift the ball up, turn it over and push it up into the sky. Separate your hands and let them float back down by your side.

Lifting a ball into the sky

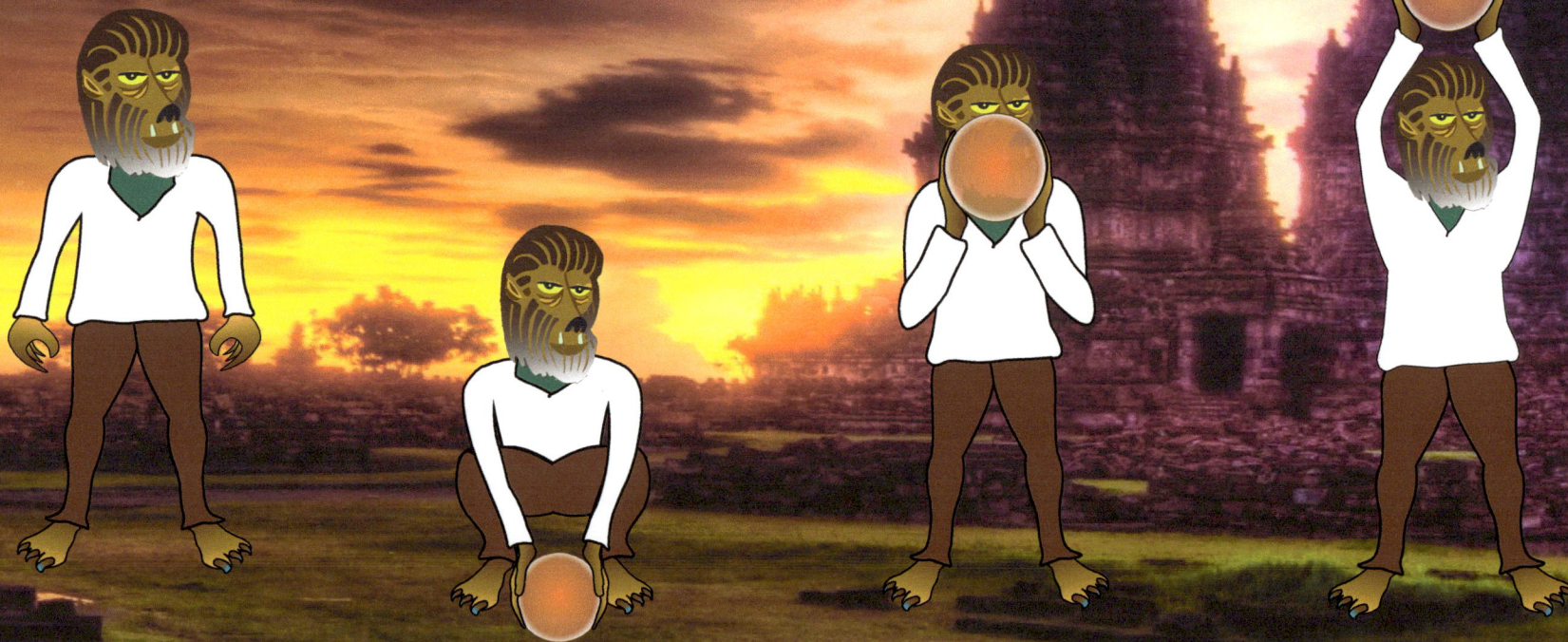

Let's try it again.
First look for the ball, reach down to pick it up, inhale and lift the ball up. Turn the ball over and exhale as you push it up into the sky. Separate the hands and let them float back down by your side. It's a simple yet very effective movement.

Try again. This time as you extend upwards think about straightening the spine. Don't overstretch just lengthen your body out. You can repeat this movement 10 times or as many as you feel you need. Each time think; long deep breaths and a slow relaxed movement.

Prambanan, Java, Indonesia.

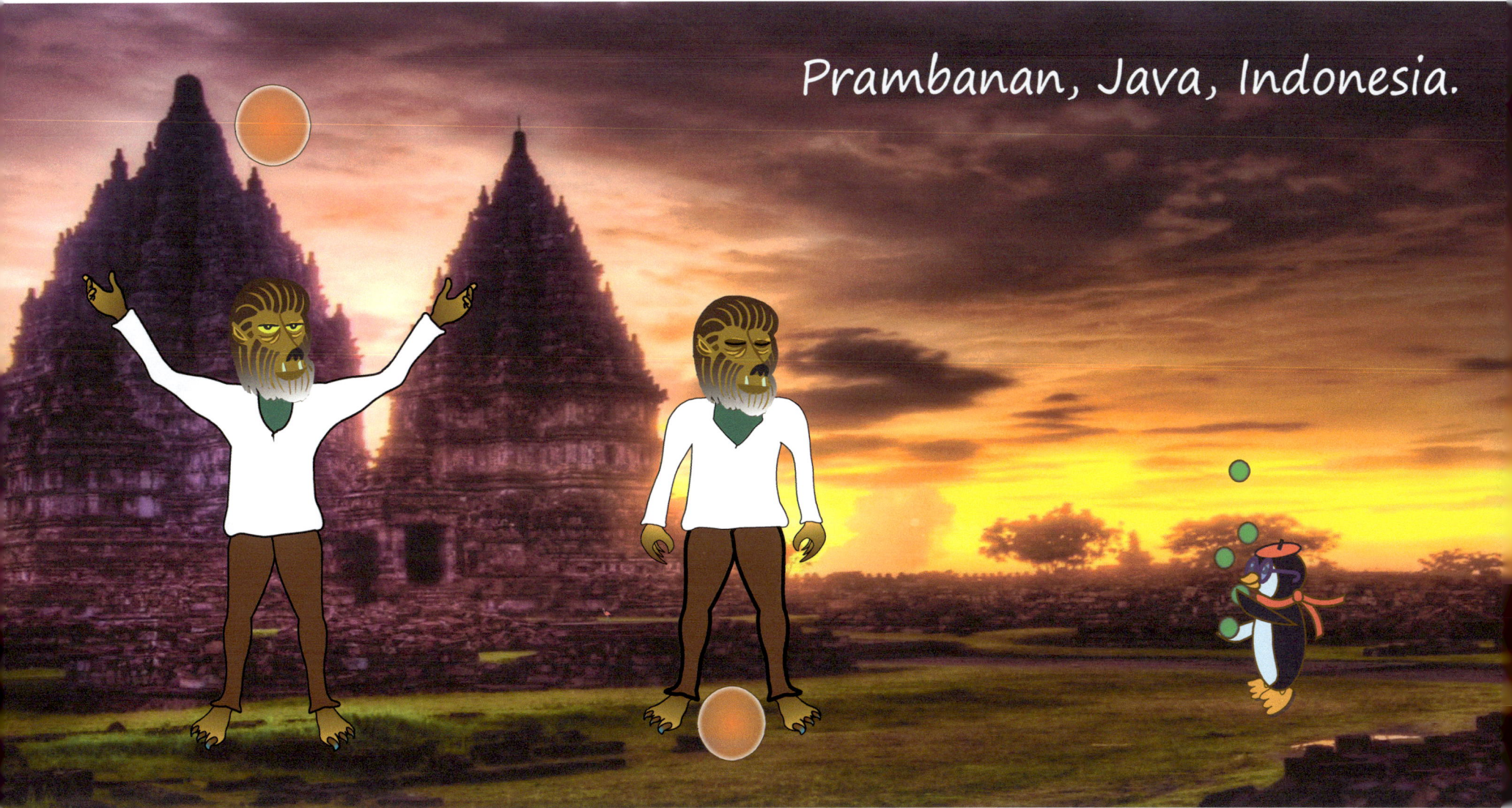

When you've finished return back to the mountain pose. Take a moment to relax and notice how all the energy you just shook up feels as it settles down. Smile to yourself and allow the happiness to flow through your body.
The previous two movements; big breaths and lifting a ball, are really good to do in the morning when you wake and in the evening before you sleep.

Floppy Twist

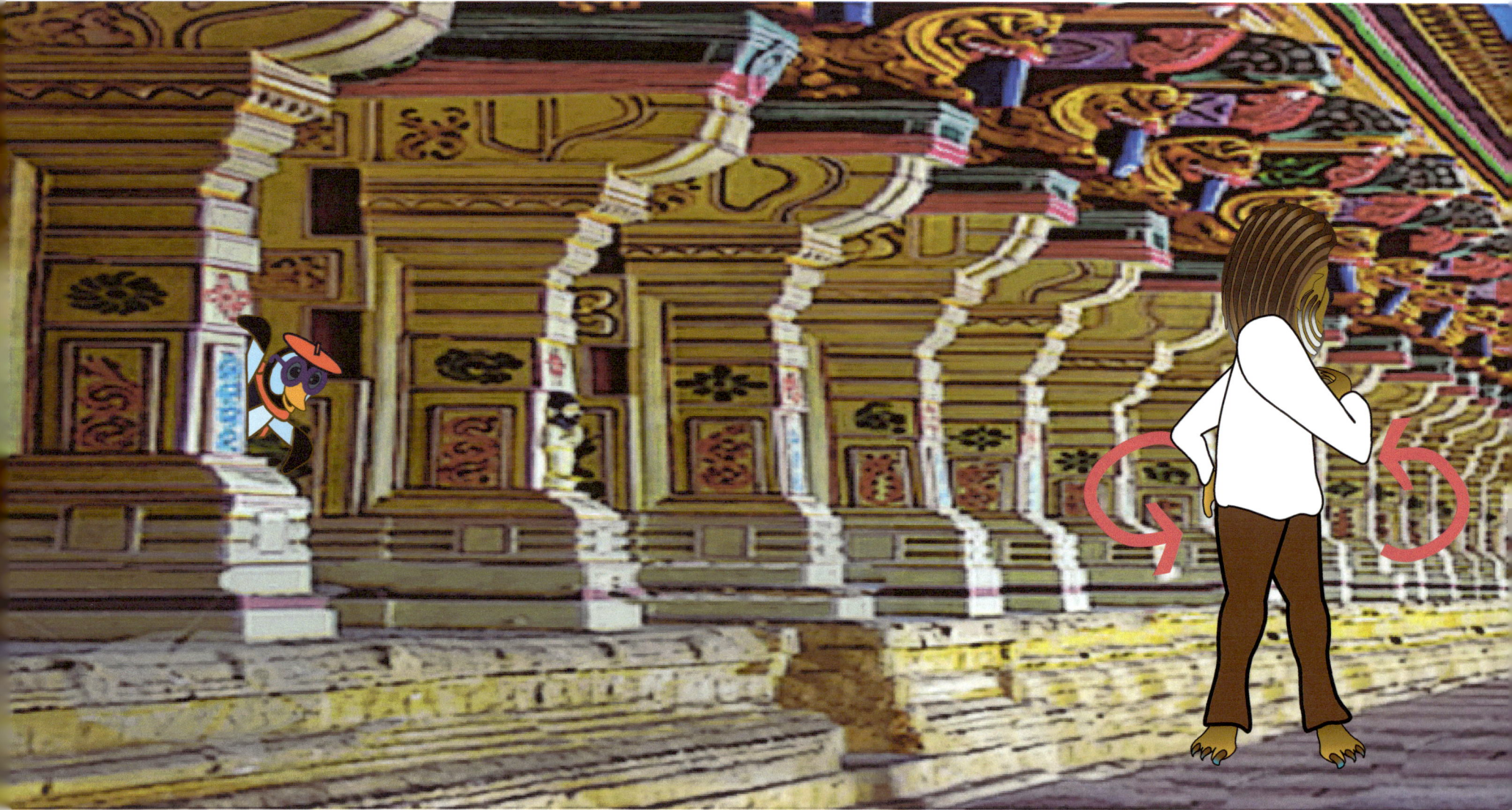

We want to think about loosening the body and letting go of tension and stress in the spine. This movement begins in the mountain pose only this time the body is soft and floppy. Keep your spine straight, the knees are soft and the arms hang limp by the sides. Begin by rotating your body horizontally, left to right, left to right around the spine. The arms will swing and flail out to the sides as you rotate. Think about smooth, slow and even rotations.

Try to find a gentle rhythm to the movement. It doesn't take much energy to move, the body is floppy and relaxed. Keep your neck soft and allow the head to fall into the rhythm, gently turning from side to side as it follows the body's rotations. Take some beautiful deep breaths and as you exhale allow the body to unlock and relax further. Remember to keep your kness nice n soft.

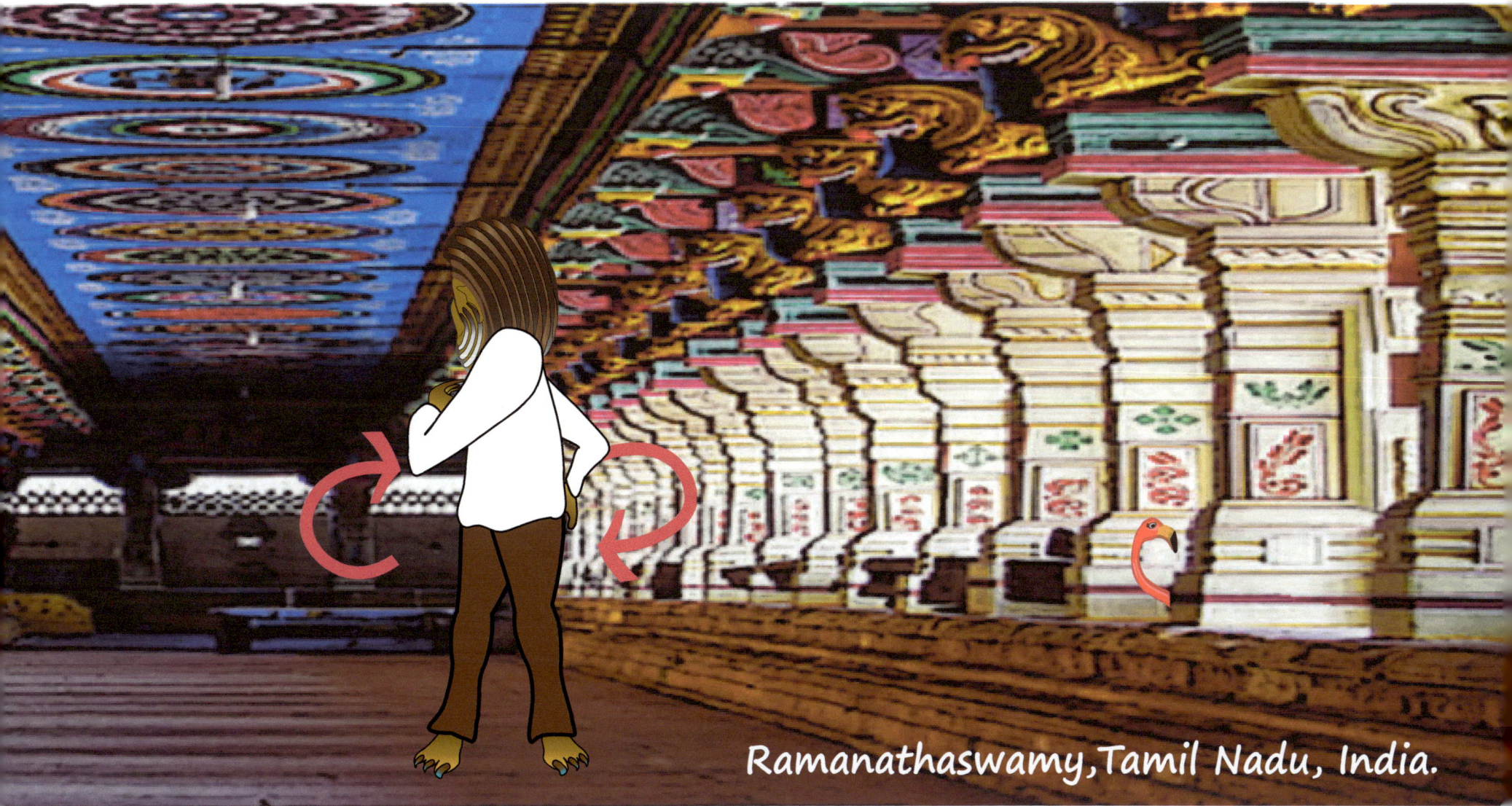

Ramanathaswamy,Tamil Nadu, India.

Keep rotating for around 2 minutes or as long as you feel is good.
When you're ready slow down and come to a gentle stop. Allow the body to relax as the twisting sensation settles down.
Take a breath, smile to yourself and enjoy the process.

We'll return now to the mountain. Take your mind down to the feet and think about grounding yourself, lift up in the chest, shoulders back, lift up from the top of the head making your spine straight, take a breath and release, feel the shoulder blades slide down your back.

Return to the mountain

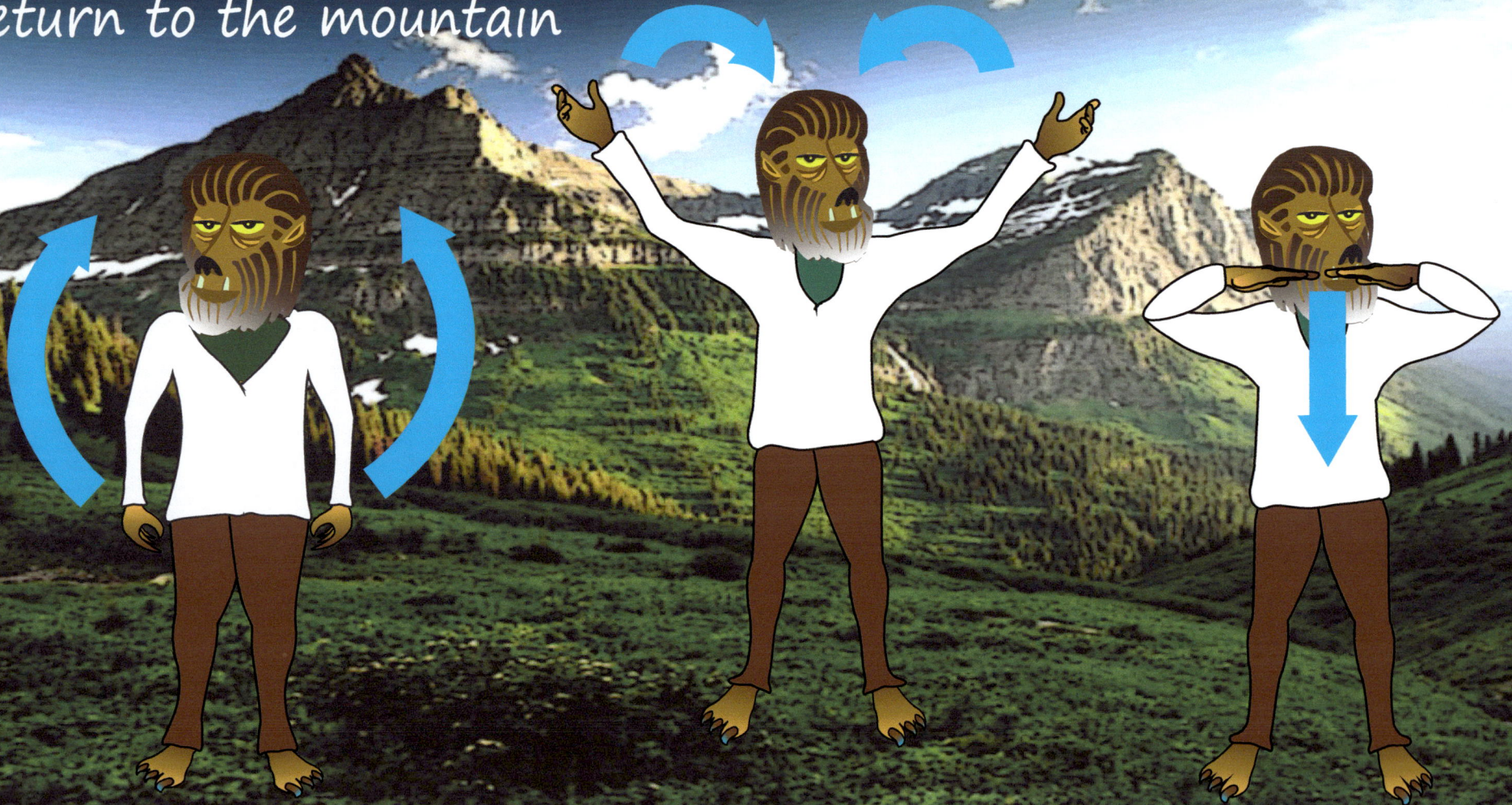

Stand up tall and proud like a mountain. The body stays up straight but the muscles soften, sinking down. Take a moment to notice how you feel. The body should feel nice and comfortable.

Let's try a few more big breaths, this time with a little difference, putting a cap on the top. Inhale and float your hands up above your head, then put a cap on the top with your hands and push the hands down in the front, keeping the palms facing down. Separate the hands at the level of your thighs and try again.

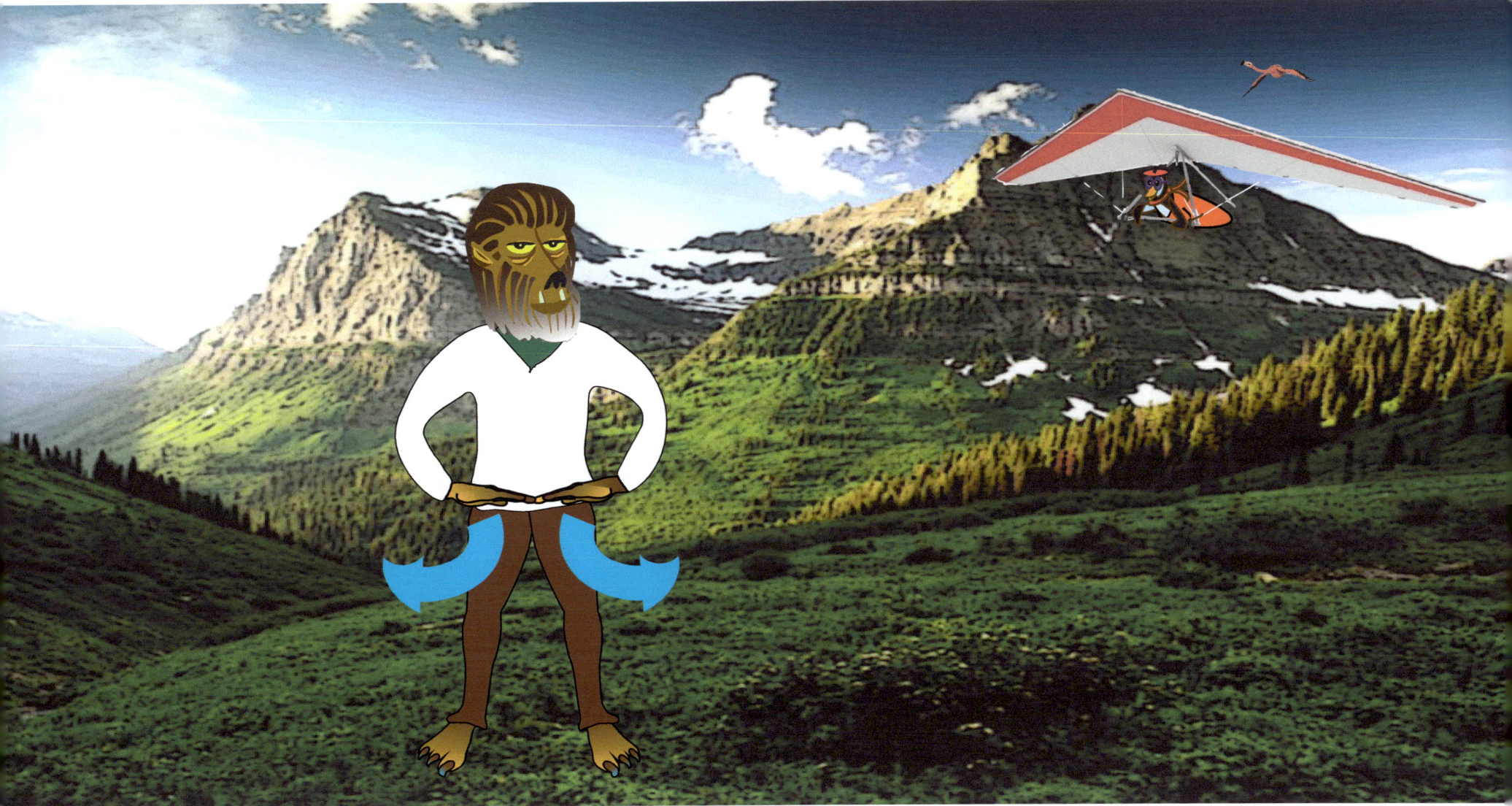

Inhale rise up, exhale float down. Repeat this move about five times. In your mind think about centring, grounding and relaxing as you float the hands down or think about returning to the mountain.

This is a beautiful movement that compliments the last. Floppy twist opens and relaxes the spine whilst the cheeky monkey deeply twists and stretches the muscles that support the spine, from the thighs and pelvis up to the neck and shoulders. Let's give it a try. Step the feet out wider than shoulders, place your hands on your knees, fingers on the inside, bend the knees and assume a squat position. Now we look for a cheek monkey.

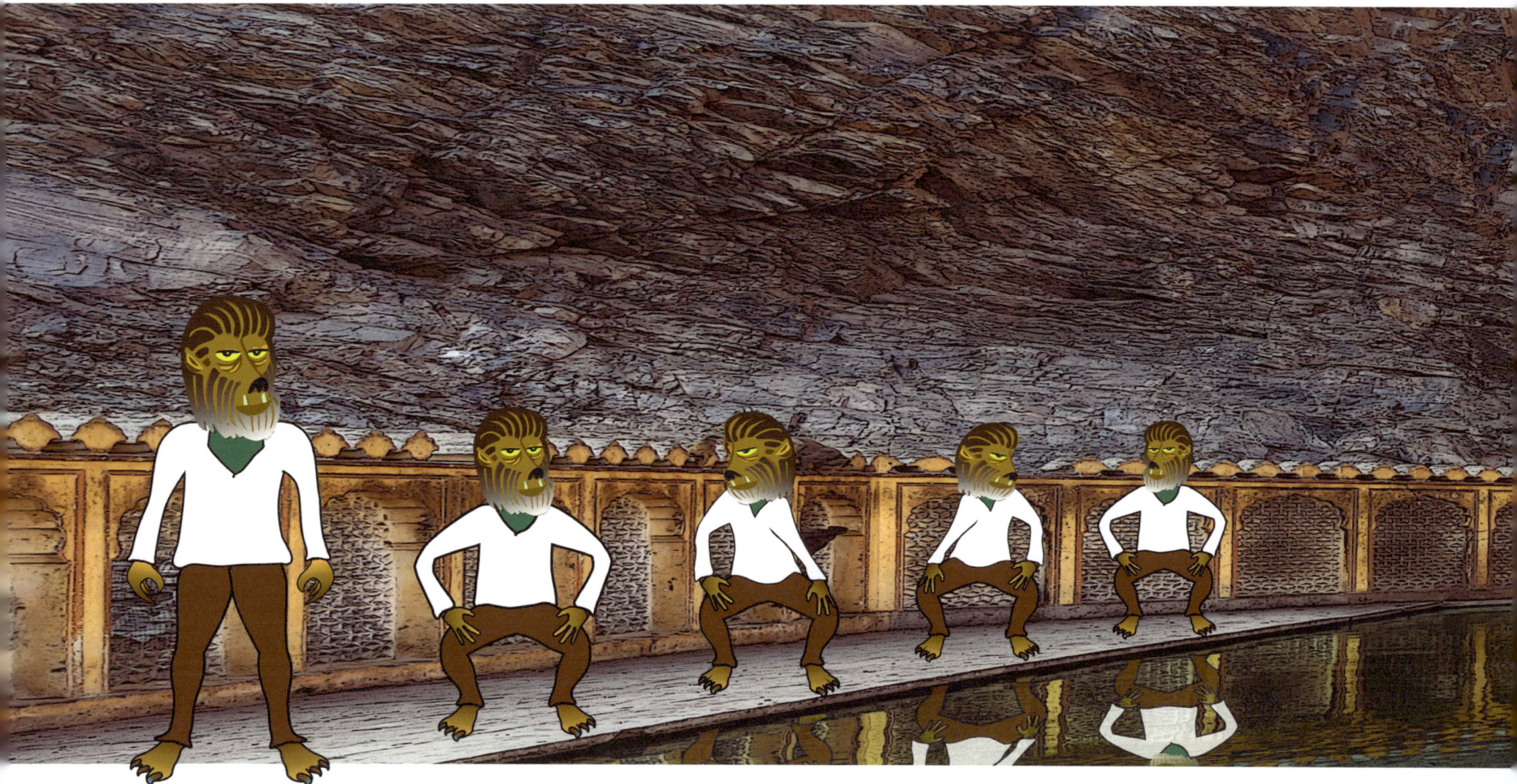

Begin on the right. Turn your head and look to the right allowing the spine to twist and follow the head. Drop the left shoulder down a little and gently push with your left arm. Take a breath and as you exhale relax into the twist. Take a second breath. This time as you exhale change sides and look to the left. Drop your right shoulder and gently push with your right arm. Take a breath and relax into the twist. Take a second breath, as you exhale change sides and look back to the right. This time turn and look behind you, twist in the spine as much as you feel comfortable and breathe. Can you see any monkeys back there?

Take a second breath, exhale and change sides, look to the left and behind you, twist in the spine and breathe. Smooth deep breaths and a soft comfortable twist. On the next exhalation change sides, looking to the right, behind you and up to the sky, twist in the spine, breathe and relax. Repeat for the left side. Take your time, relaxing into each twist. As you come back to the centre take a breath before standing up.

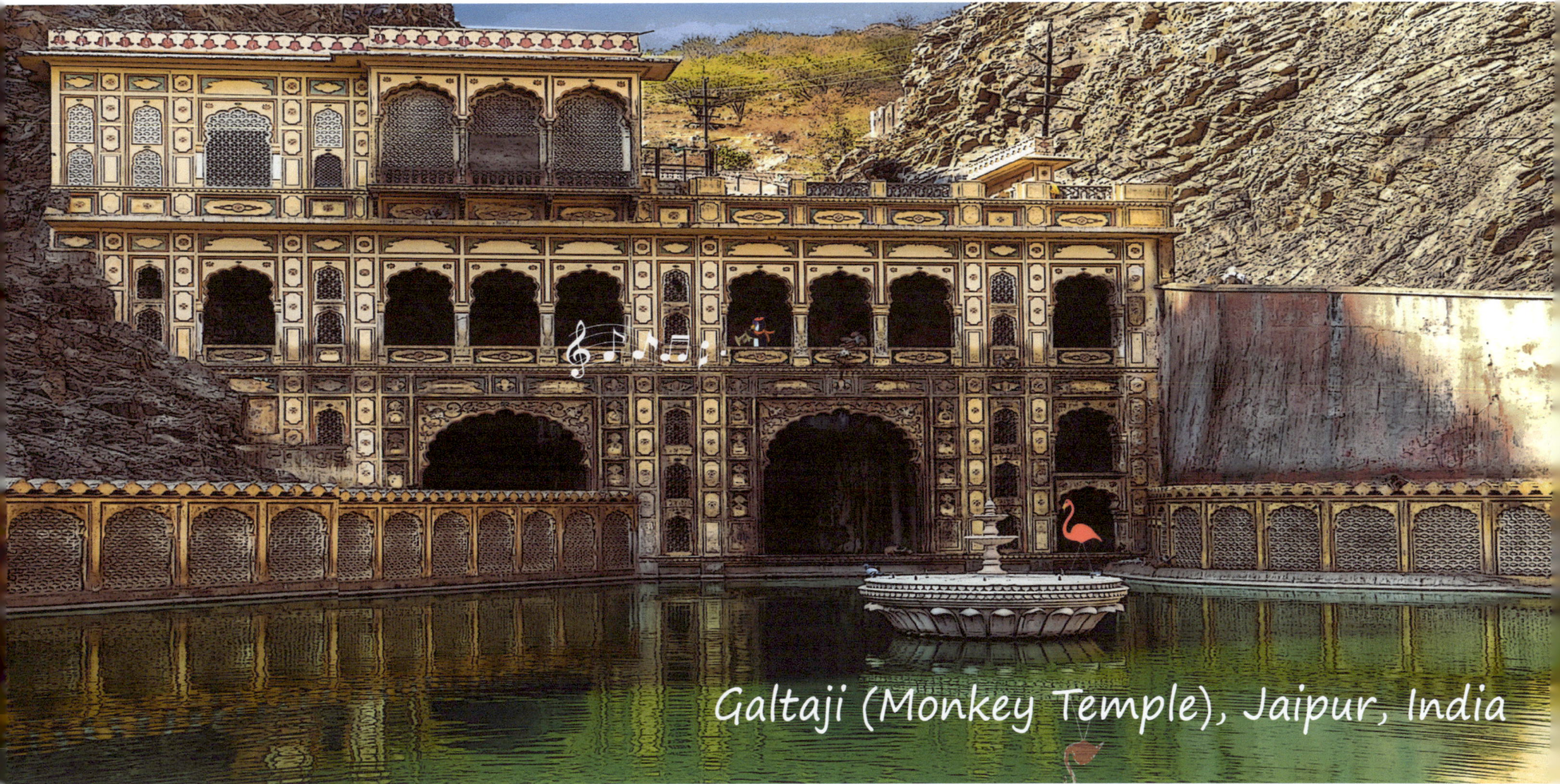

Galtaji (Monkey Temple), Jaipur, India

Step the feet in and return once again to the mountain. Find your centre as you breathe and relax allowing all the energy we shook up to settle down. Take a moment to smile to yourself. When you smile to yourself you make a happy positive connection with your body. If you walk down the street and smile at someone they smile back and you both feel good. It's the same with your body. Smiling to different parts of your body helps them to feel happy. Remember your body is your friend, when we smile at our friends we all feel good.

This is a classic move that proves itself time and time again; year after year it's so good for you and so easy to do. I'm sure you have done it many times before but perhaps never consciously.

Hip Circles

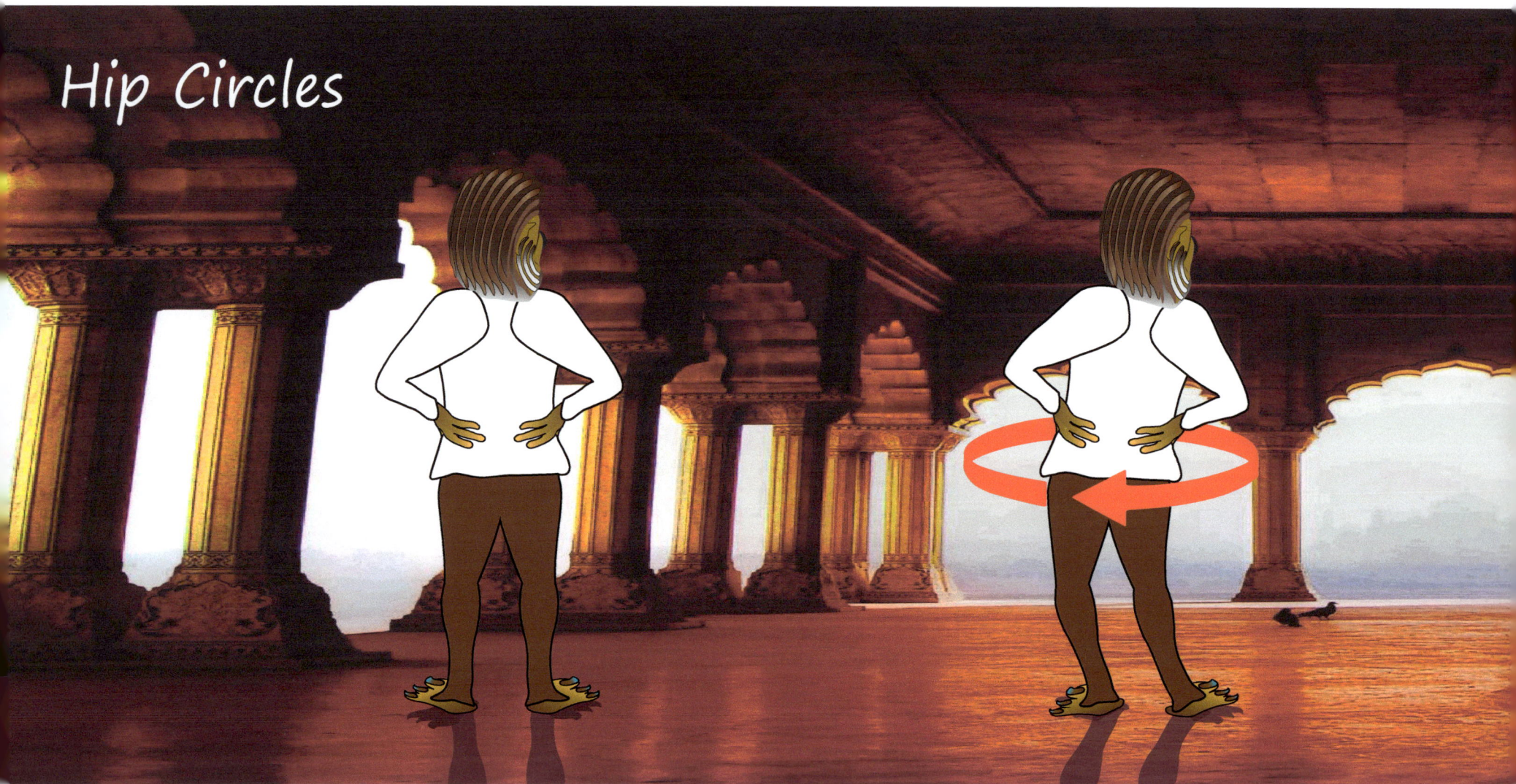

Begin in the mountain pose, your feet about shoulder width apart. Place your hands on the lower back, fingers in towards the spine and the thumbs facing down. Point your elbows backwards. Rotate the hips in a clockwise direction about 5 times and then reverse the move for 5 times in the other direction. Think about pushing your hips to the outside of the circle. Take a deep breath and relax into the rotations.

Take your mind down to the pelvis, Feel the muscles and bones that are involved in the movement. Take a deep breath and in your mind try to lead the oxygen down to your pelvis to nourish and enrich the area. As you exhale breathe out any negativity or tension that you may feel. Remember to relax, take it slow, smooth and easy.
Take a moment to smile to yourself and enjoy the process of rediscovering your body.

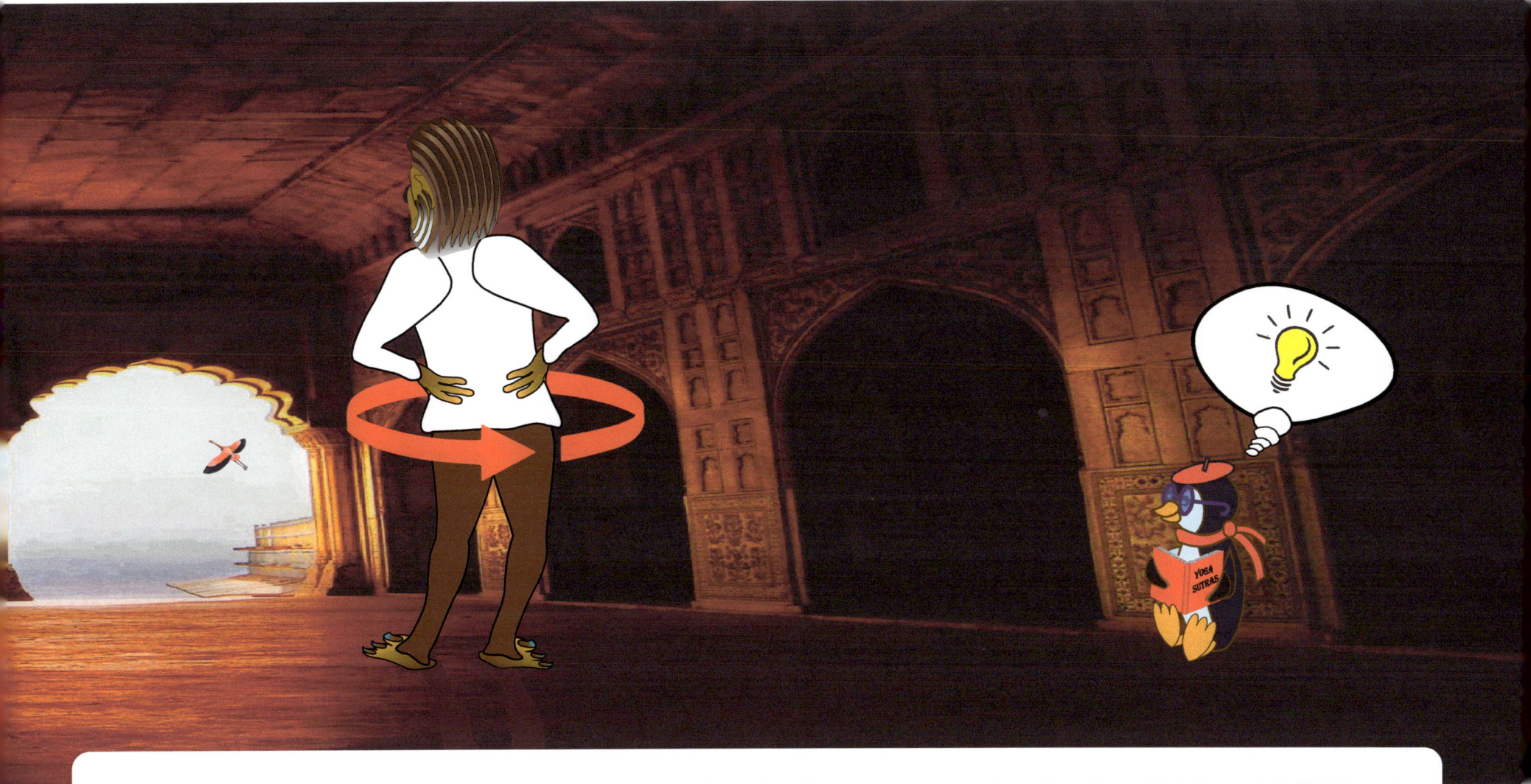

   In yoga we put our body in different positions; we breathe then we assess the situation. Did it work? Did it not work? Which muscle groups am I targeting? Which bones are being manipulated? Does it feel good? How does my breath feel? What thoughts are in my mind? You don't have to answer these questions, just become aware of them without judgement. Not good or bad, just aware. As we relax into various postures we learn how to open the body and how to get the breath to flow to different muscles, organs and bones.

Most of the problems in the human body are inside the head or psychological. Brain cells use about ten times more oxygen than normal cells. I believe it is the lack of fresh blood supply to the brain that causes most of these problems. Inversions are an important part of yoga and there are many ways to do them. An inversion is when we take the head below the heart. All of the fresh oxygen in our blood will flow into the head, refreshing the brain. When is the last time you inverted your body?

Uttanasana – The Forward Bend

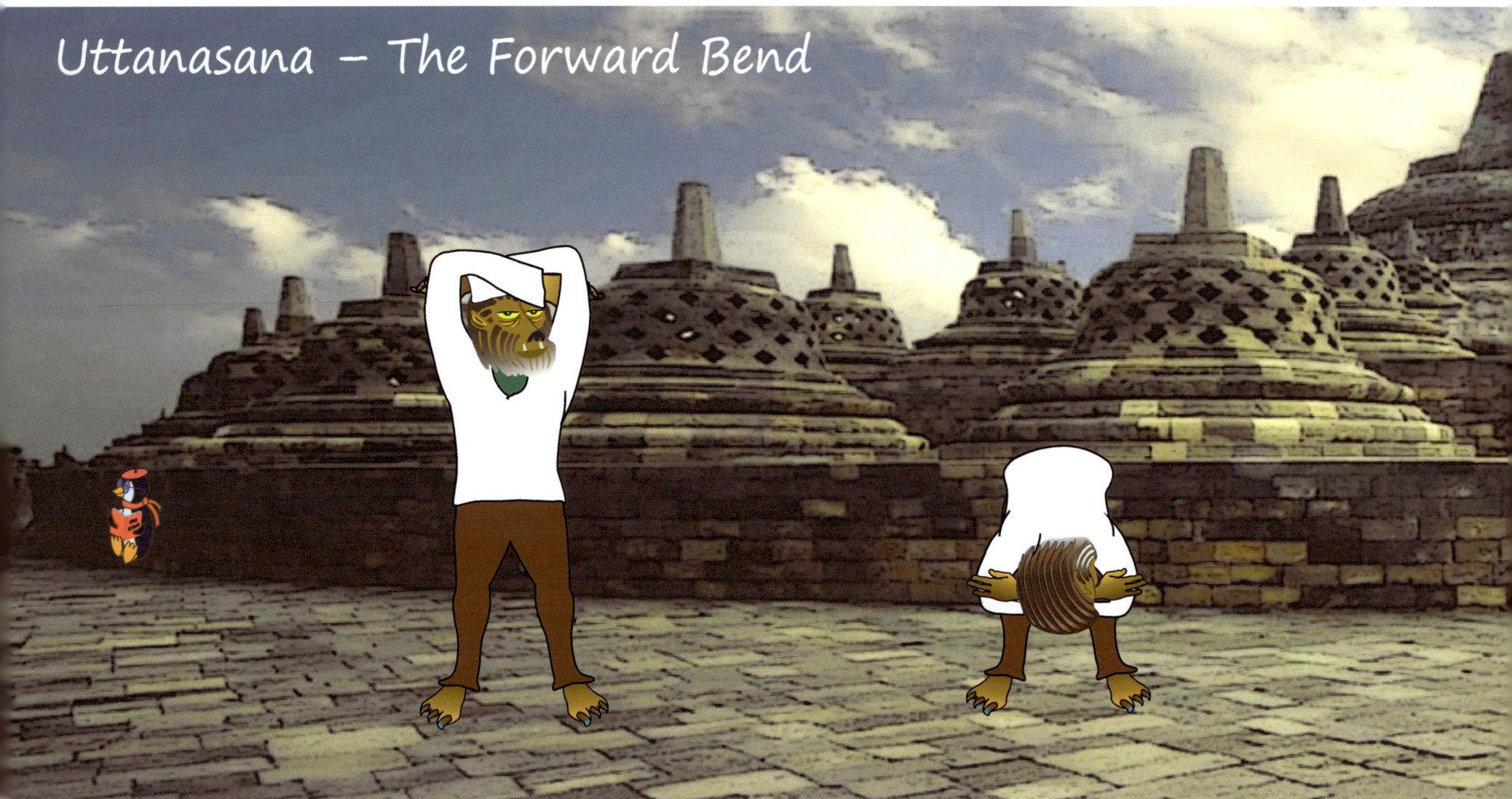

If you think about it the average person never inverts their body. They wake up in the morning and move around all day with the head never going below the heart. Even when they sleep the head is elevated on a pillow. I believe this lack of oxygen to the brain causes many untold problems. An easy way to begin fixing these problems is to invert the body.

This asana is really easy and has many health benefits. We'll begin in the mountain pose: tadasana. Float your hands up above your head and take a deep breath. Cross the arms then slowly fold forward. Keep the legs straight and let the weight of the arms hang down. That's it! It's very easy. Now just simply hang out here and breathe, exhale and relax into the posture. Shake the head from side to side to release any tension in the neck and focus the mind on the breath. With each exhalation the body relaxes and becomes soft. Stay here for about 5 breaths.

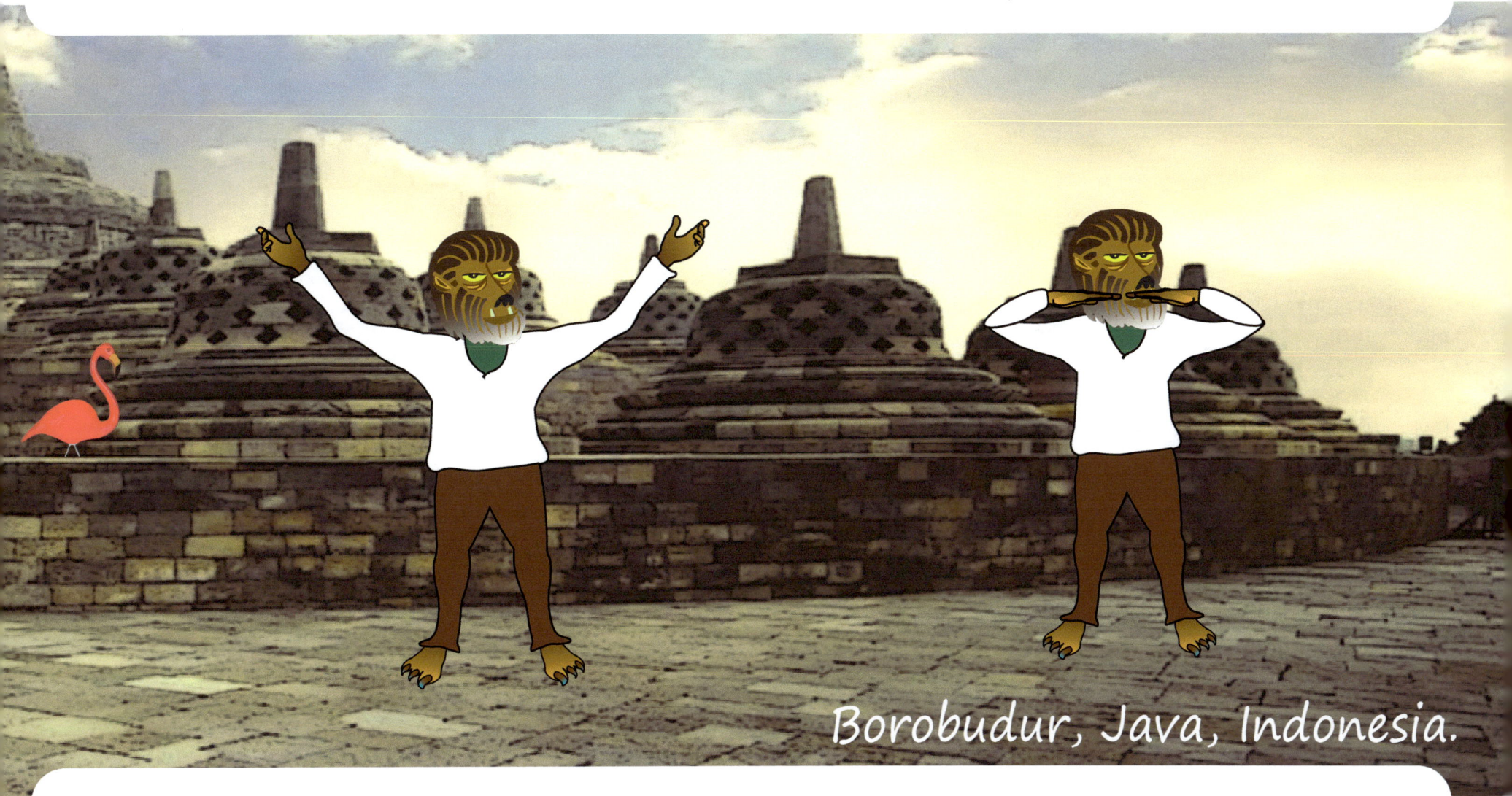

Borobudur, Java, Indonesia.

Imagine yourself as an elephant. Let your arms sway a little, maybe a few centimetres each side, just like an elephant's trunk. Breathe and relax. To come out of the pose, exhale, soften the knees, release the arms and slowly rise up. Inhale as you float the hands up above your head, place a cap on the top, exhale and pull down in the front. Return once again to the mountain. Allow all the energy you just shook up to settle down.

Breathe and release that which no longer serves you.

The breath is our welcome into this world. Exhaling and breathing our last is our exit. If we cut off the air supply the body will die in a few minutes. If you breathe too deeply the muscles become tense and stressed. If you breathe too little the body will start to shut down from lack of oxygen. For something we do every day and don't really think about, it's pretty important to get it right. Most people have no idea about the breath and its value for the body. They only consider it when it becomes short, like when we climb stairs or go for a run. The reality is that the human body runs on oxygen; the brain, the muscles, the bones, the organs all need a good supply to keep them operating properly. Lack of oxygen will severely deplete their ability to function at a normal level, on the other hand if we introduce more oxygen into the system, it will   function more efficiently.

The body is designed to process things; foods, thoughts, emotions, feelings, air and liquid and eliminate the waste products from the system. The more efficient the waste disposal is, the cleaner and healthier our body will be. Constipation and other problems caused by toxins not being removed is an extremely important topic in the yogic scriptures. If we don't eliminate waste products, they will accumulate and be a breeding ground for bacteria, sickness and eventually pain. For example, every day millions of blood cells are born and millions die. This waste has to go somewhere. Spent cells are turned into carbon dioxide and expelled through the lungs. The lungs and our breath are the first line of offence in removing toxins from the system.

The body eliminates toxins and waste in three ways. The first is via the lungs, which regulate oxygen levels and remove a large amount of gases and pollutants; the second is via the kidneys, which process liquids; and the last is via the intestines, which process more solid matter. These friends do all the hard work in removing the crap that we put into our bodies every day: bad thoughts, bad food, bad water, bad air and bad feelings. Day after day the organs labour intensely to process our bad decisions. Toxins that are not processed get stored in the body and eventually create problems.

It's time to give the body a rest!

If we could turn just one of the bad things into something good, we could enjoy amazing results.

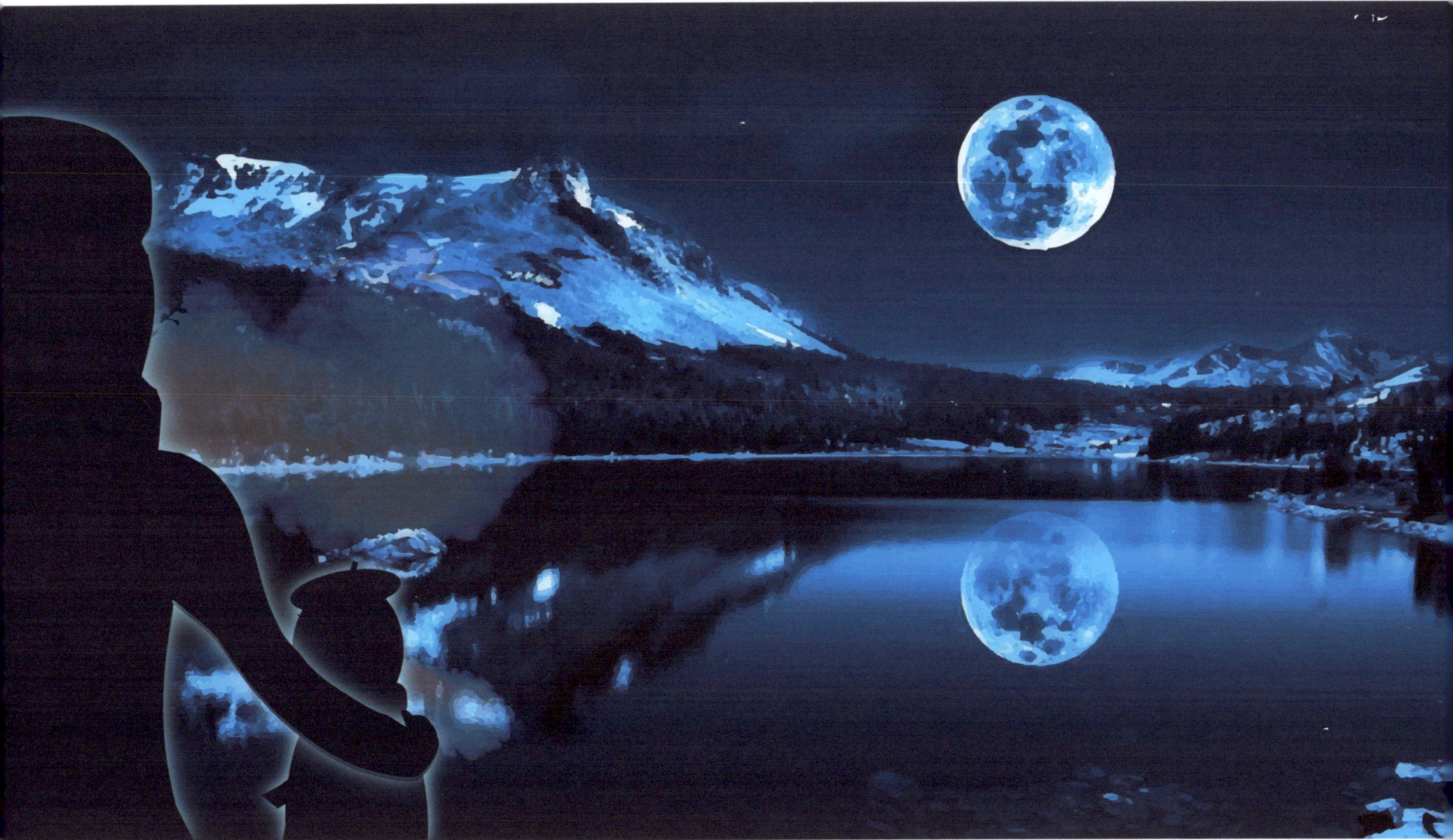

We could breathe more, drink more water, stop allowing emotions to affect our thought patterns, and we could think more about the quality of the food we put into our body. Very easy stuff to consider yet people go on struggling with no hope in sight.

Let's think about water for a moment. Some people don't drink it, ever!

They drink coffee, beer, soft drinks and so much other stuff but never plain water.

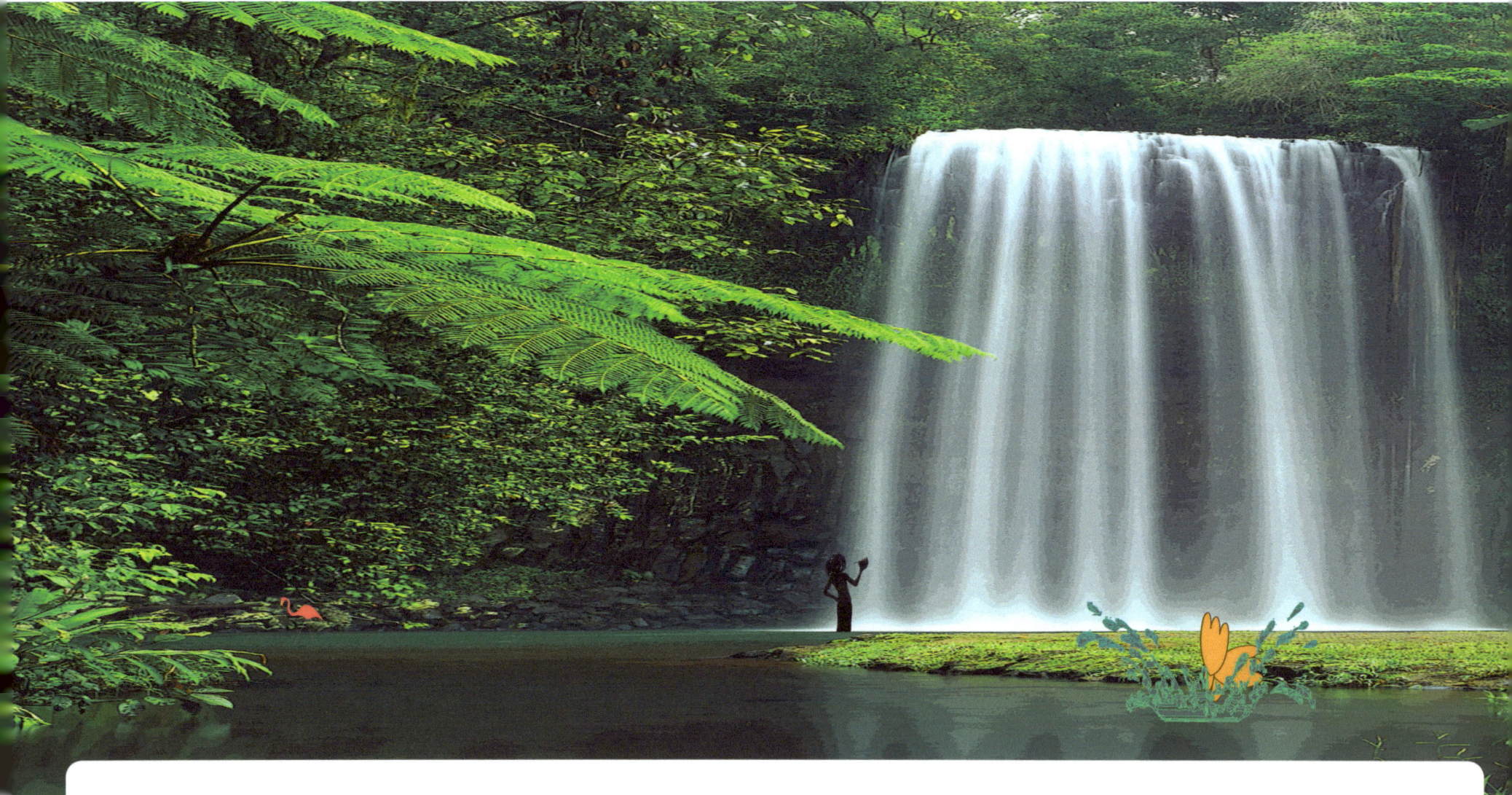

Our body is made of more than 70% water. It's always processing liquids and expelling them from the body. We need to replenish this loss of fluids with fresh, clean water. Our kidneys need water to flush toxins from the body. If we only drink fizzy soft drinks, the sugars and acids they contain will build up in the body; we won't get rid of them. The kidneys will be overworked and will become sick or simply fail and if your kidneys fail you're going to be in a world of pain.

So what do most people do?? They drink more coffee, more beer, more fizzy bubbly and put more pressure on their kidneys to perform. They need a rest! Give them some fresh clean water, the best you can afford. If we keep topping up the system with new water, the toxins become diluted and are easily flushed from the body. The muscles and organs become lubricated and function at their optimum level.

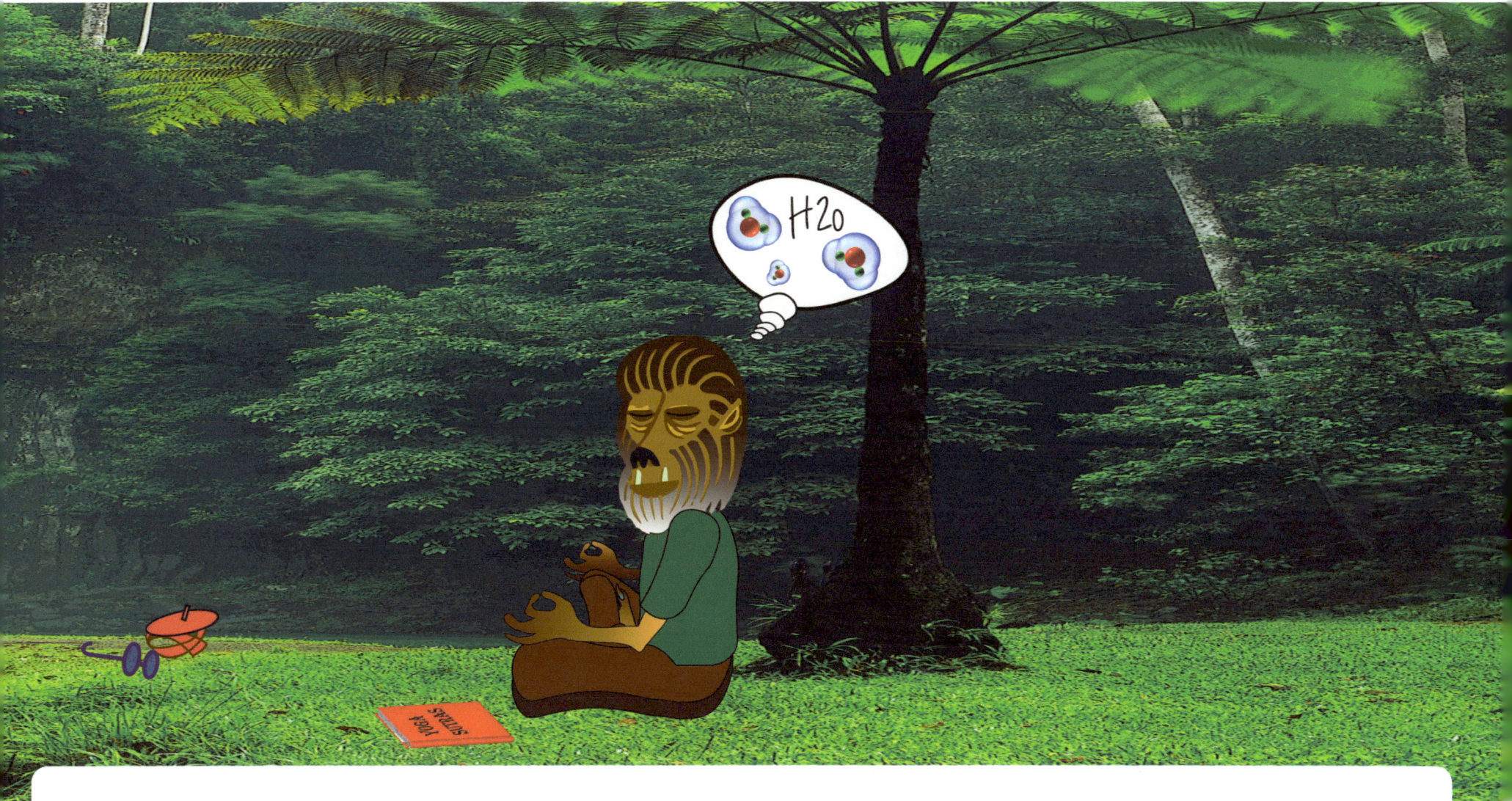

You can see from this simple example just how important good quality water is. I recommend a glass a day for the beginner. Just one glass, it's so easy, you can drink it in ten seconds. Give it a try. For the person already acquainted with water it's time to up your dosage; one, two or even three litres a day will really hydrate your system and help you to feel happy and revitalised. For the professional; you already know this so keep up the good work.

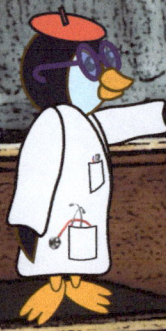

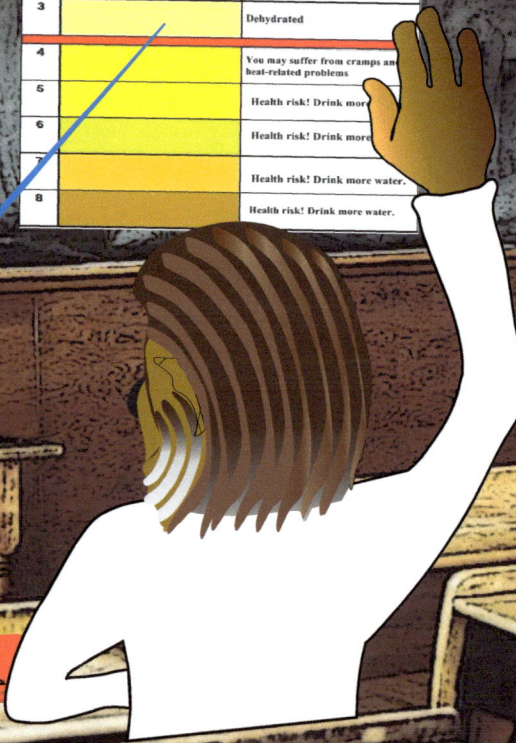

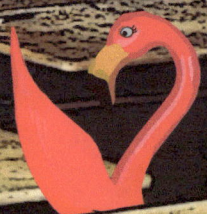

Thoughts to consider:

1)   Observe the colour of your wee. A clear or light yellow colour means the metabolic or growth processes are functioning properly. A darker yellow and sometimes even orange colour means that the catabolic or decay processes are functioning properly. Do you want to encourage growth or decay inside your body?

2)   Due to our modern diets, the body has become way too acidic. An acidic body that regulates at 37 degrees is a prime breeding ground for bacteria and sickness and more often than not cancer. One way to combat this is to flush the system with water. Another, much more effective way is to neutralise the acids with an alkaline substance. I recommend Apple Cider Vinegar with the mother. Take a tablespoon mixed in a glass of water every day, in the morning, or in the evening, or both. This will have a positive effect on the acids in your body, neutralising them and rendering them harmless. If we neutralise the acids then the liver and kidneys don't have to work so hard to eliminate them. Also, modern enthusiasts say that cancer will not grow in an alkaline body. But don't take my word for it! This is a prime situation for independent study. If you choose to research these topics I'm sure you'll find people much more qualified than me who will confirm my statements.

3)   Your body is designed to poop every day to remove waste products from the system. This is a normal function. Some people only poop once a week. This is abnormal. The waste products build up inside the body putting extra pressure on the organs. Under pressure the waste sticks to the walls of the intestines and bowels and hardens making it more difficult to remove and becoming a breeding ground for bacteria and sickness. If your poop is hard and difficult to pass out, this means you are dehydrated. Drink lots of water, it will soften the stool and help to flush the waste from your body.

4)   Get yourself a water bottle. It doesn't need to be cool or funky it just needs to be clean and be able to hold water. Now take it with you wherever you go and enjoy a mouthful every fifteen minutes or so. Hydrate the system and feel your health improve. You may need to go to the toilet more often, but remember that every time you do you are flushing toxins and waste products from the body. Think of a river. If the water keeps flowing bacteria doesn't have a chance to grow. But when the water levels drop, pools begin to form which become stagnant breeding grounds for funky stuff. So keep the water flowing. A flowing river is a happy river and brings life to the surrounding area.

There are many things that flow like a river inside the body; blood, water, energy, waste, information, vitamins, minerals and hormones. These rivers flow throughout your body. If they can flow unobstructed to their ends; hands, feet and head, then they will nourish all the different parts along the way. If they don't flow properly then you will have problems.

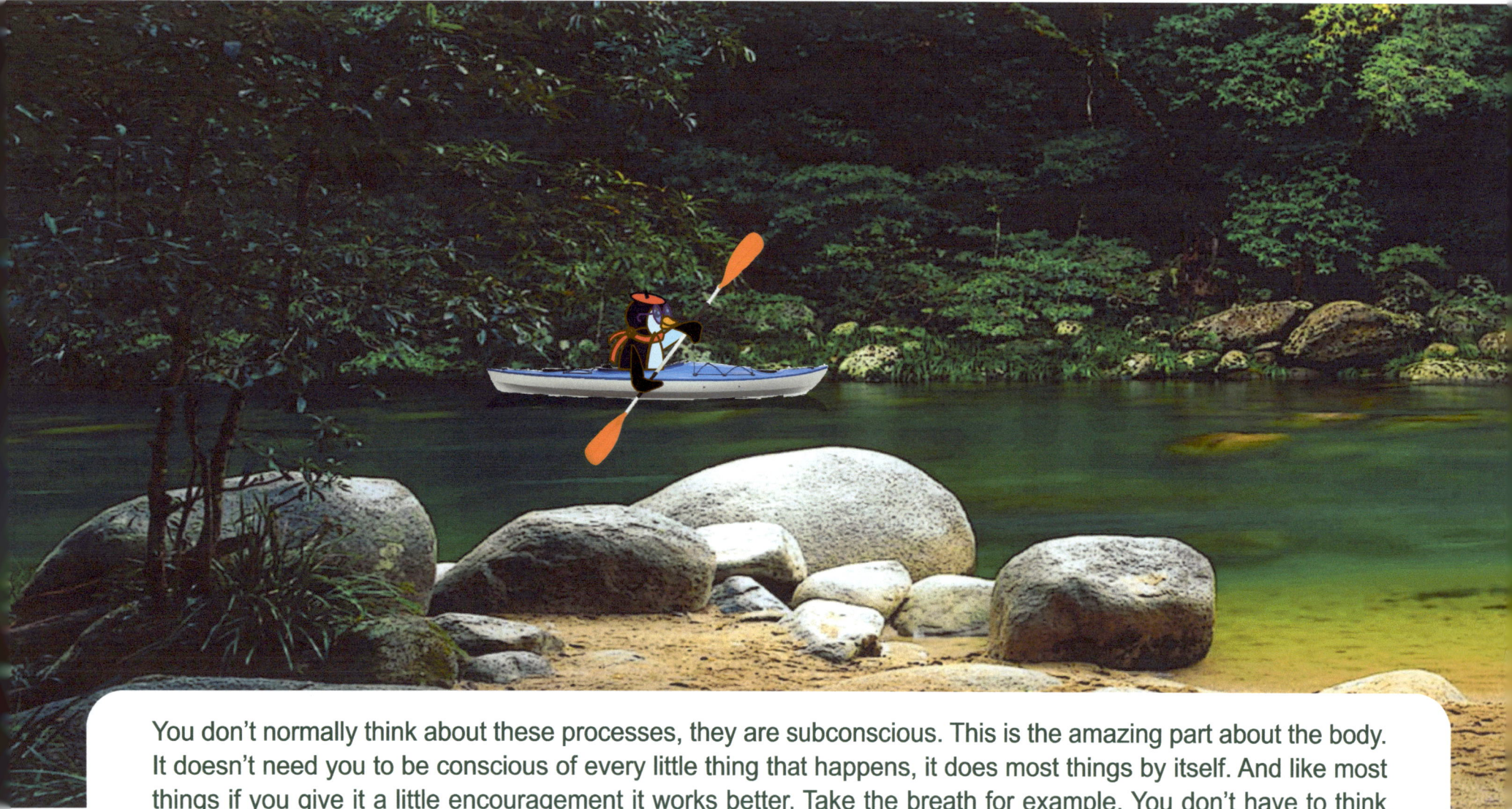

You don't normally think about these processes, they are subconscious. This is the amazing part about the body. It doesn't need you to be conscious of every little thing that happens, it does most things by itself. And like most things if you give it a little encouragement it works better. Take the breath for example. You don't have to think about it, you just breathe. You can however use your muscles and your mind to alter the breath or change the flow of the oxygen river. You can make it slower, deeper, more relaxed, more shallow, faster or you can even reverse the flow. You can also lead the breath to different parts of your body for nourishment. In the same way you can use your muscles and your mind to alter the flow of other rivers in your body.

Think about your hands. If you hold them together, rub them or clap them what happens?
They become warm. How?
You used your muscles and your mind to generate blood flow to this area.
It's the same for all parts of the body.

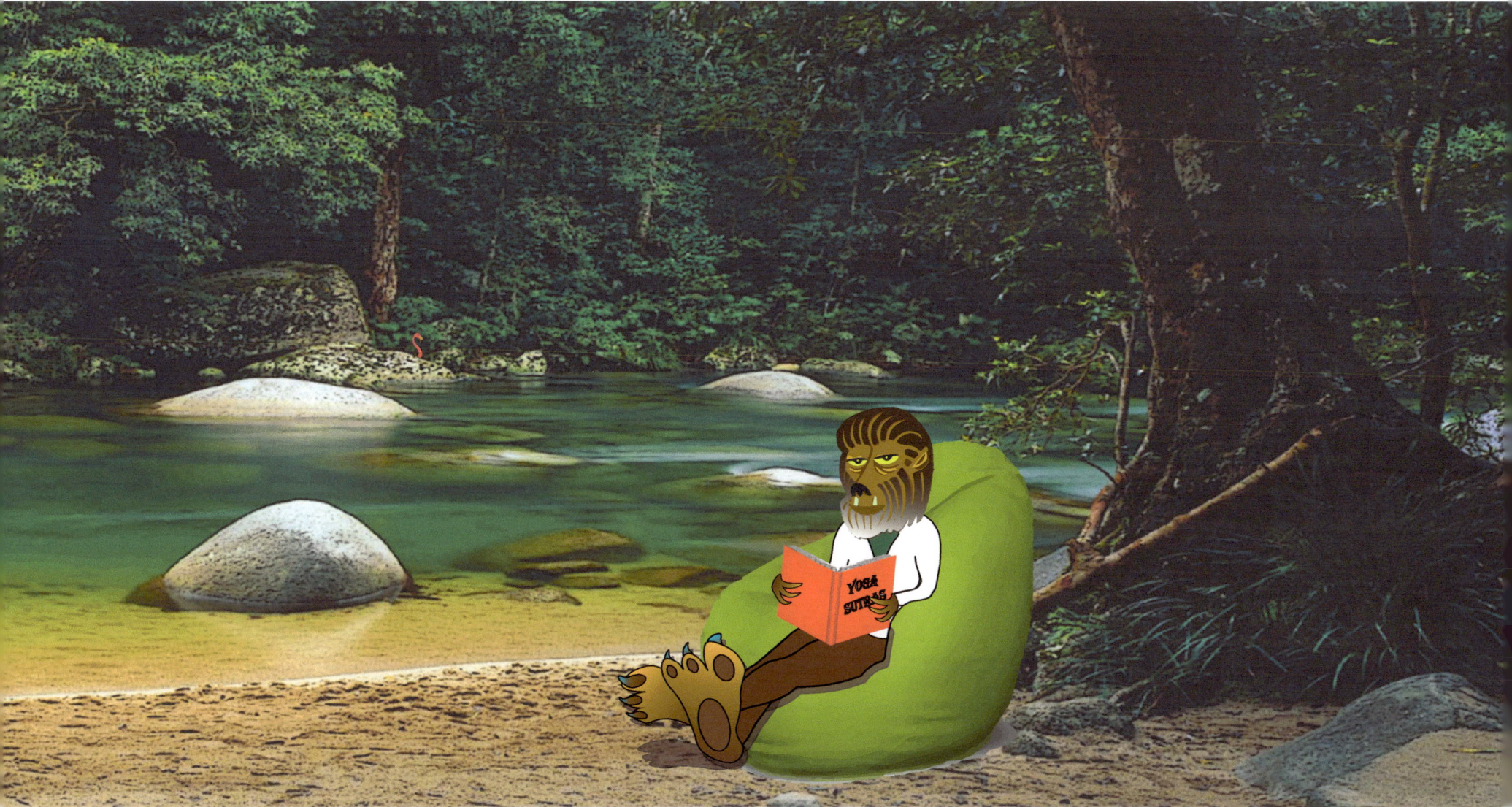

Your blood caries oxygen, vitamins, minerals, bioelectricity and other goodies to nourish and heal all of the cells in your body. It also takes the waste products back to the lungs where they are expelled with the breath. So by this rationale if we stimulate the blood to flow more, it will work more efficiently.

Let's start tapping all over our body, just a general tapping to stimulate the whole system. Fast or slow, it doesn't matter just tap tap taparoo. All over the body are hundreds of acupressure points, when you tap, you not only stimulate these points but you also promote blood flow. If the blood can flow to the extremities; hands, feet and head, it will nourish all the organs and muscles along the way.

Tapping

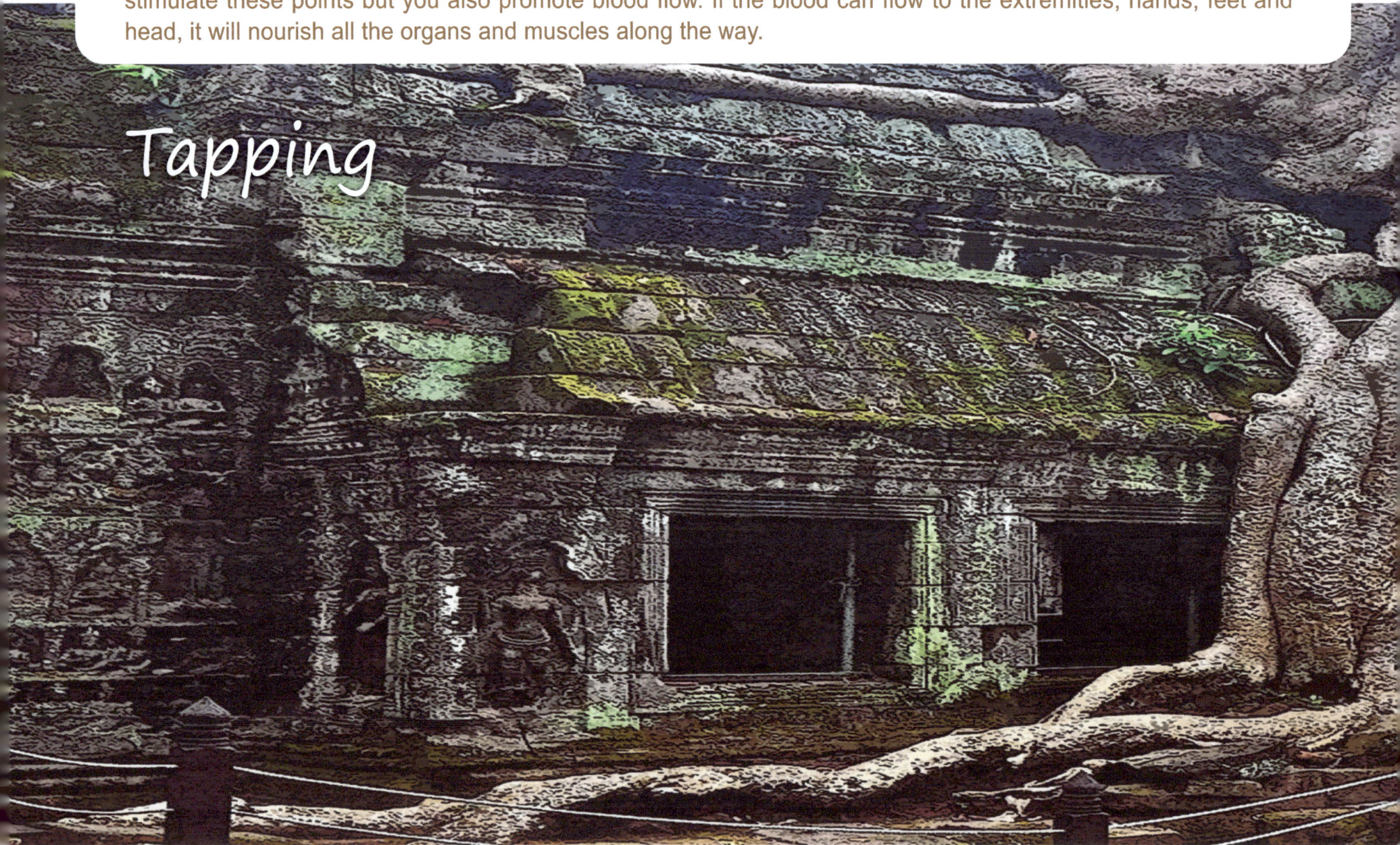

Take 5 – 10 minutes to tap and awaken your whole body. In your mind think about the blood flowing to all the places you tap. Refreshing and rejuvenating, carrying away toxins, opening up blockages, nourishing and cleaning. Take some deep breaths and enjoy the process.

When you tap you don't want to hurt your body, you want to stimulate blood and energy flow. It's your body so you know how hard to tap. Take it easy, smile to yourself and have fun.

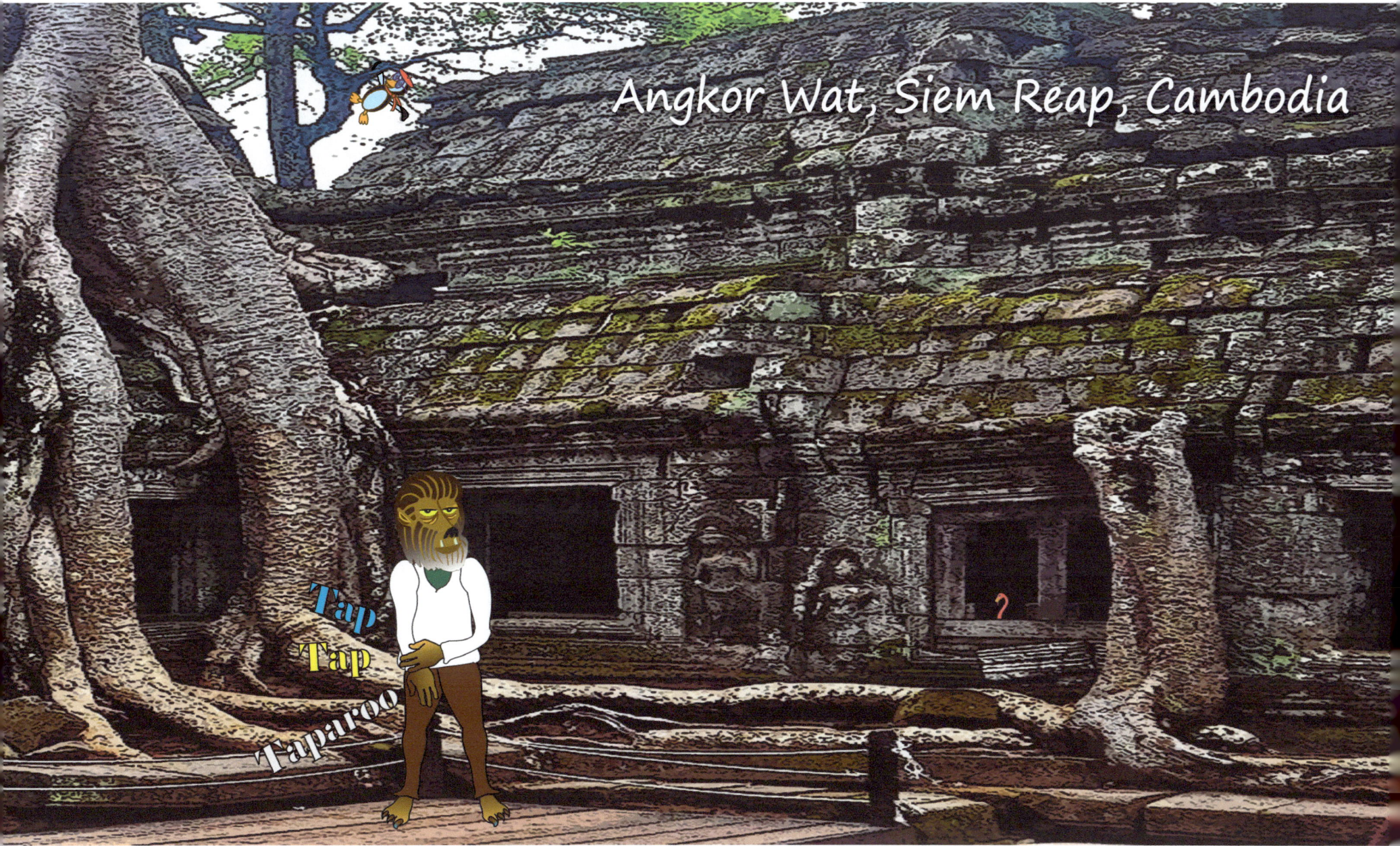

Angkor Wat, Siem Reap, Cambodia

Tap
Tap
Taparoo

When you finish, return to the mountain. Let all the energy you just shook up, settle down. Notice how it feels. Breathe, relax and enjoy the sensations. Take a moment to smile to yourself. Feel the happiness and good vibes growing and expanding inside of you.

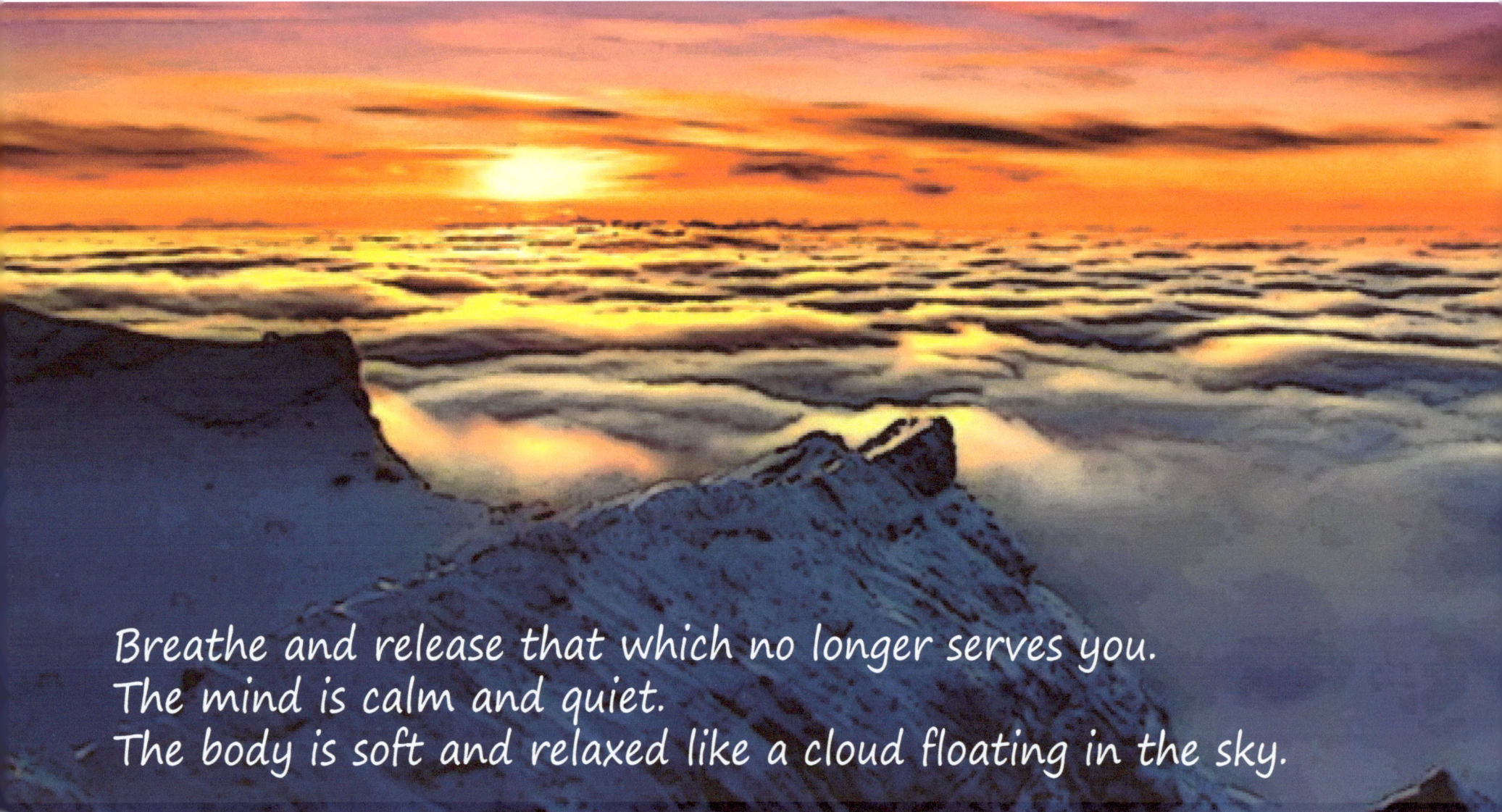

Breathe and release that which no longer serves you.
The mind is calm and quiet.
The body is soft and relaxed like a cloud floating in the sky.

Next bring your awareness to the tip of your nose and become aware of the breath there. You don't have to look at your nose – just put your mind there and notice what happens. Breathe in through the nose and breathe out through the nose. What can you feel? Try again and see if you can feel any difference between the in and the out breath.

Did you feel it? The 'in' breath is cool and the 'out' breath is warm. This is how your nose filters the air that comes into your body. Next try to feel where the air goes to inside of your body. Take a deep breath and follow it with your mind. Where does it go to? Which part expands?

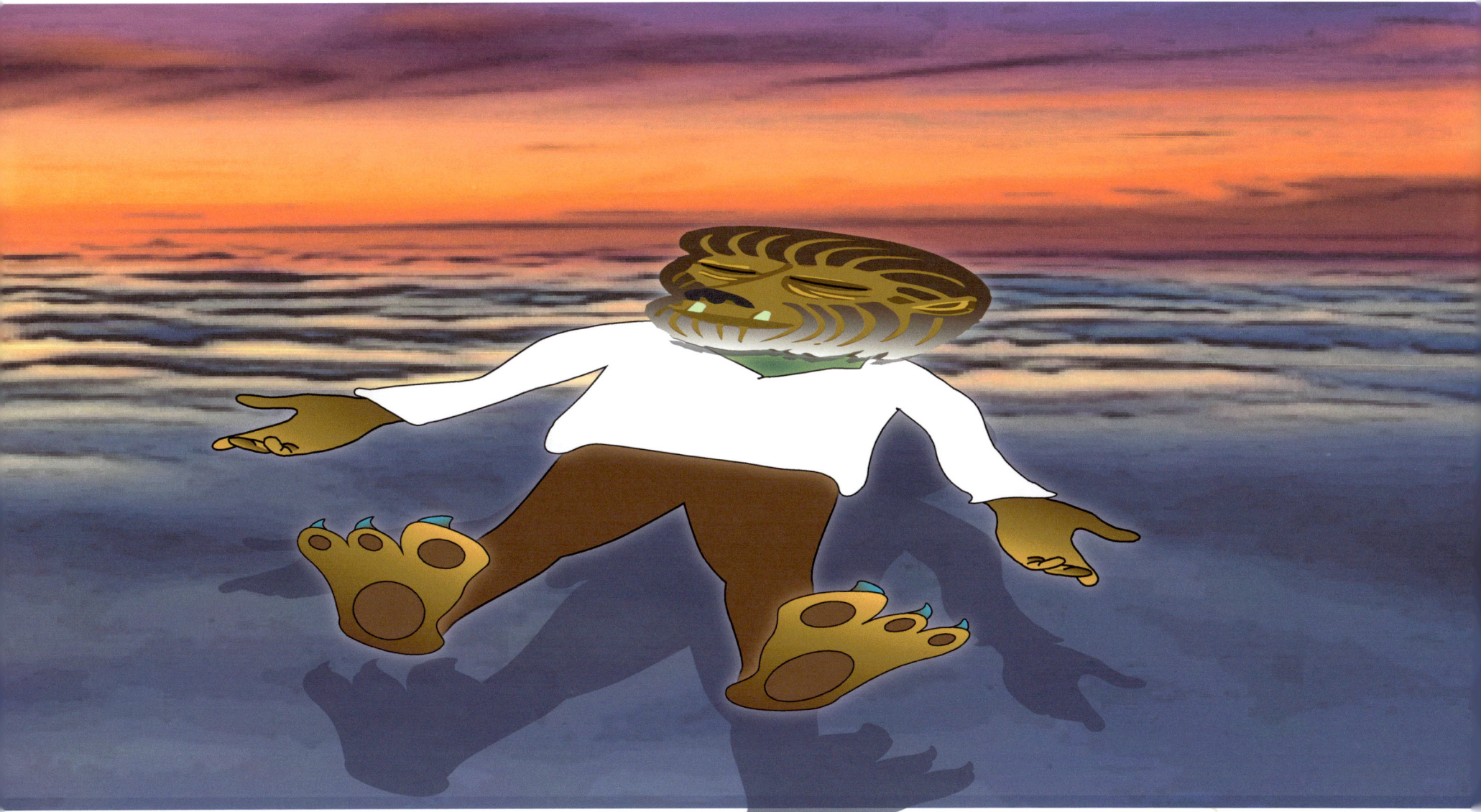

Now breath out, follow the breath back up and out through the nose. Which part of the body contracts as you exhale? Try again and see if you can feel it.

If you felt your chest expand and contract this is called thoracic or chest breathing. It's usually quite shallow breathing and doesn't bring much oxygen into the body, however it does energise the body. We breathe like this when the body is cold, tense, angry, nervous, excited or anxious. It is characterised by a 'flight or fight' state of mind where the body is not comfortable so it tries at all costs to protect itself by energising.

Breathing

Diaphragm

Chest Breathing

Belly Breathing

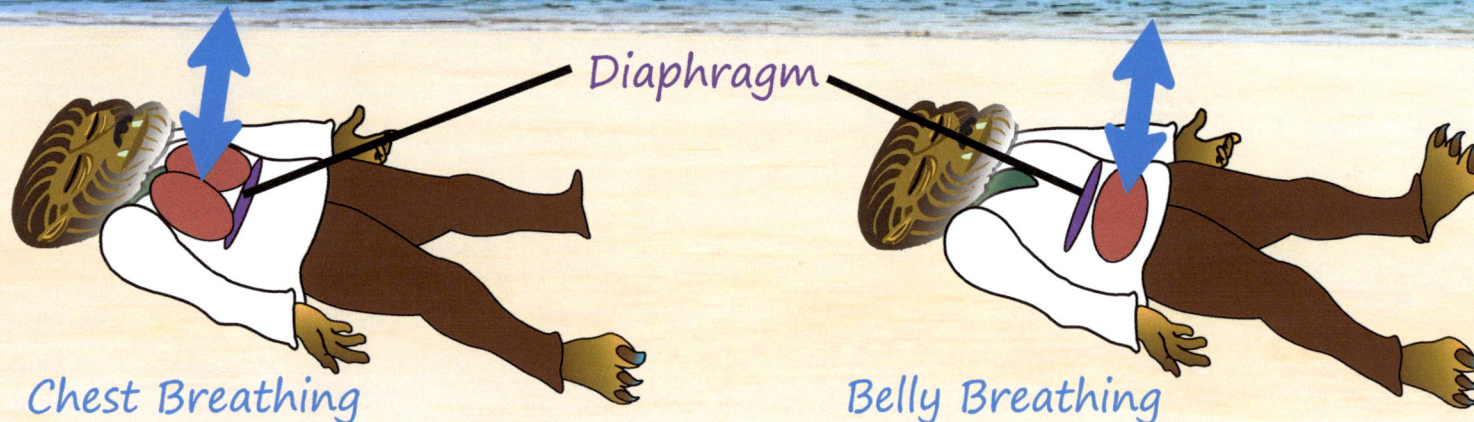

If you felt your belly expand and contract then this is called diaphragmatic or belly breathing. It's a mid-range breath and brings a good deal of oxygen into the body. The diaphragm is located horizontally in the body at about the level of the lowest ribs. It acts as a pump to bring the oxygen into the body.

If the diaphragm moves down, oxygen flows in and if the diaphragm moves up oxygen flows out. This is considered normal breathing and is characterised by a 'rest and digest' state of mind. In rest and digest the body is healing itself. The mind is calm, the body is relaxed comfortable and the organs can function at an optimal level.

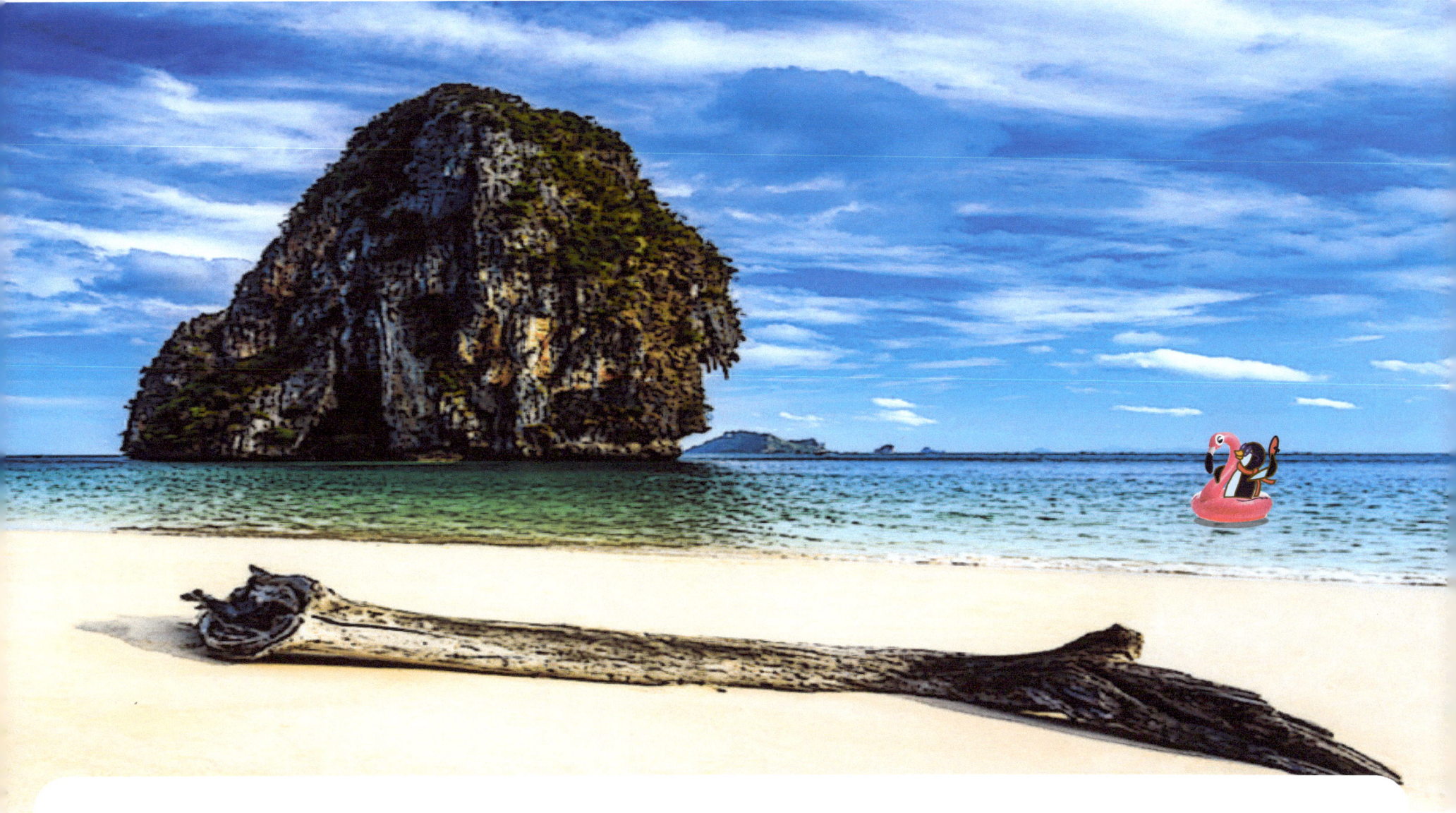

When we think about the breath, we think about leading it deep into the body to maximise oxygen absorption. The more oxygen or life force we bring into the body, the better it will function. This life force is called Prana and it is directly proportional to the breath. The more we inhale the more prana or life force we gain.
Breathing exercises are called Pranayama.

To breathe, first you must breathe out, creating space for the incoming breath. Use your abdominal muscles to push the used air out of your body, then simply relax and let your body fill up with fresh air. Lead the air or prana with your mind, in through the nose and down deep into the belly, allowing your belly to expand. Next relax and feel the used air flow up and out of your body. Again use your abdominal muscles to push the last bit of used air out. When all the air is gone, relax your abdomen and inhale filling up your belly again with fresh prana. Then relax the belly and let the used prana flow out again.

Try 10 breathes like this. Don't strain your abdomen just relax into the breath allowing it to flow naturally. When your mind wanders consciously bring it back to your breath. Inhale. Belly expands, lungs fill with air. Exhale, belly contracts pushing the air out of the lungs. The spine is straight, the body calm and relaxed. Focus on your breath and the sensations it generates within the body. Think about making your breath slow, smooth and slender.

This is considered normal breathing. If it feels uncomfortable it's because you have been breathing wrong your whole life. Nobody ever teaches you how to breathe or how to walk for that matter, you just learn it for yourself. Young children breathe like this naturally but due to fear and anxiety in their lives, a fight or flight mindset is generated and shallow breathing results. This is a learned behaviour or a bad habit which I believe causes many problems later in life. A big part of yoga is unlearning all of the bad habits which you think are good for your body and replacing them with the truths you'll find through regular practice. The truth is that lung capacity is nearly 6 litres. The average human breath is about 300 – 500 mls, less than 10%. Is it any wonder that we have problems when the body clearly doesn't get enough oxygen?

Most people never consider the breath until it becomes restricted and even then they don't think about it as we are now. The study or science of the breath is called Pranayama. One of the main reasons we practice yoga is to fill the body with prana. A body abundant in prana does not get sick or degenerate like other bodies do.

Relax your breath now and just let it return to the normal breath for your body, notice how it feels. Take a moment to enjoy the sensations generated inside and outside of your body. Begin to wiggle the toes and the fingers drawing the awareness back into your muscles. Bring the feet together, take the arms above the head and have a nice big stretch. Roll onto your side and come up to a sitting position.

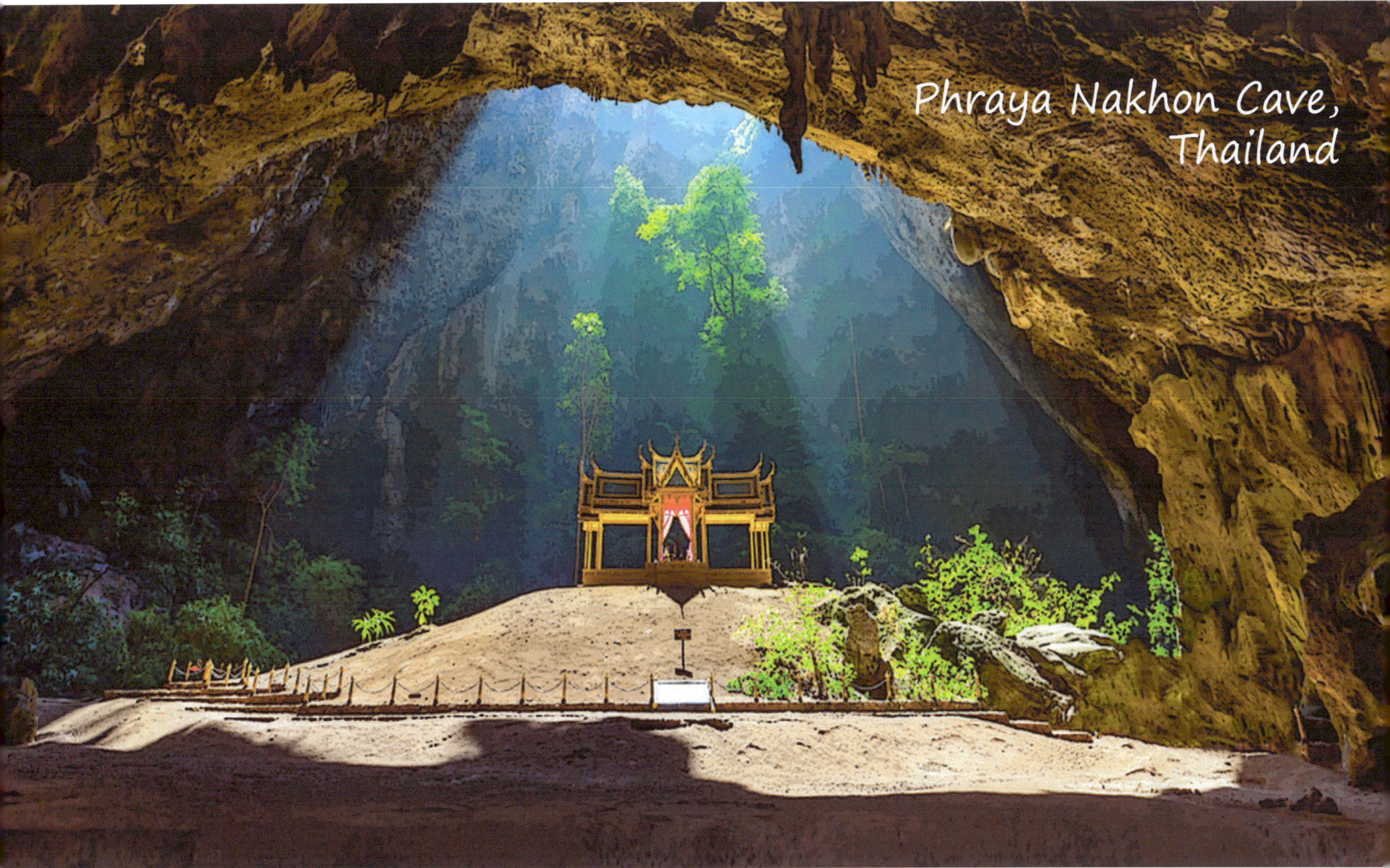

Badhakonasana – The Butterfly

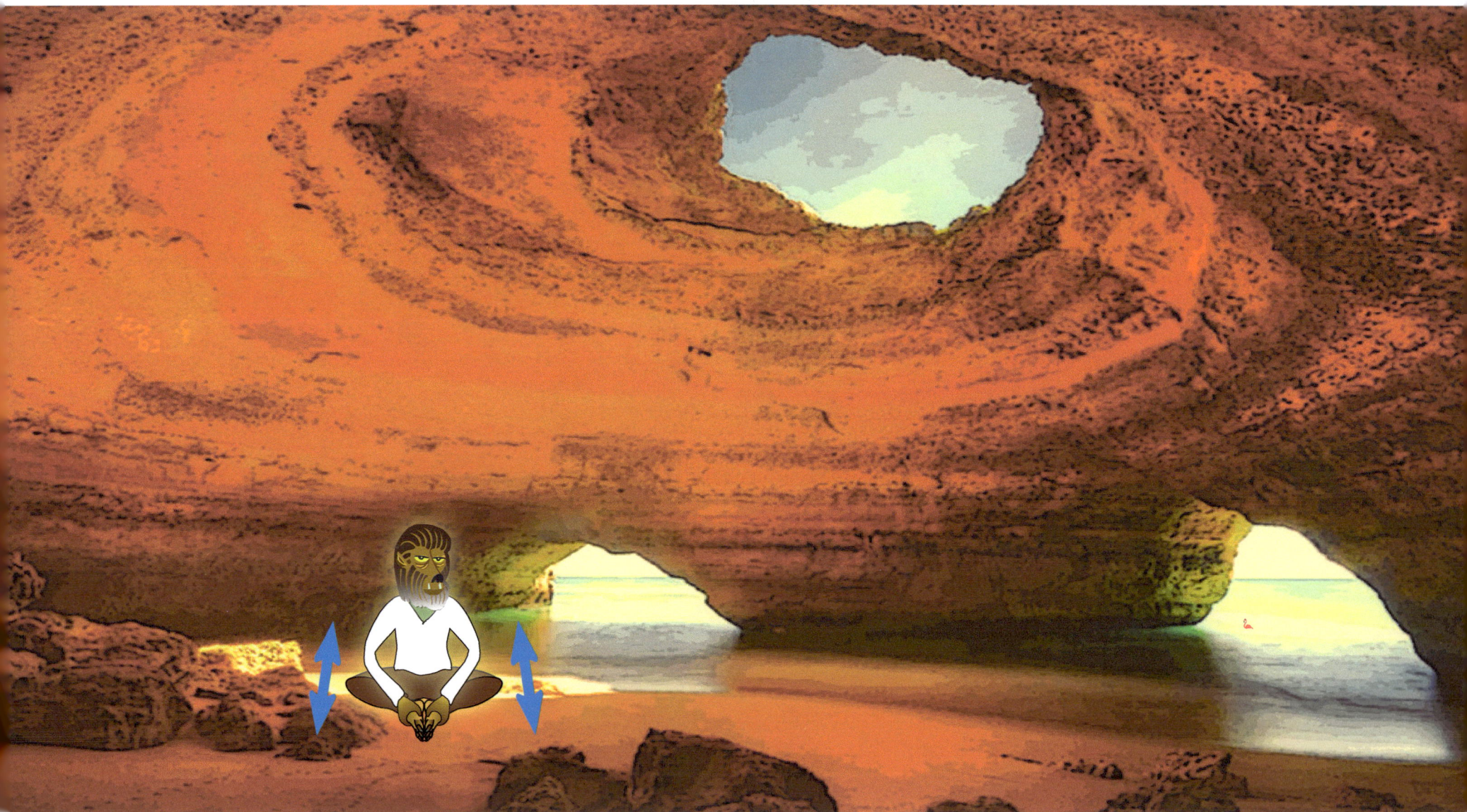

Let's try some butterflies. This is such a beautiful move to open and relax the pelvis. Bring the soles of your feet together, hold onto your toes with both hands and draw your heels in toward your groin. Next rock your knees from side to side, one knee up, the other down, alternating between sides. Take a breath and relax into the movement. Think about leading the breath down into your pelvis.

Sea Cave in Benagil Beach
Algarve, Portugal

With each exhalation consciously open and relax your pelvis. Lift up in the chest and keep your spine straight. This is our first variation. Keep rocking from side to side. The second variation is to rock both knees at the same time. Take a few minutes to explore each variation, breathing and relaxing into the movement.

Sukhasana – The Easy Seat

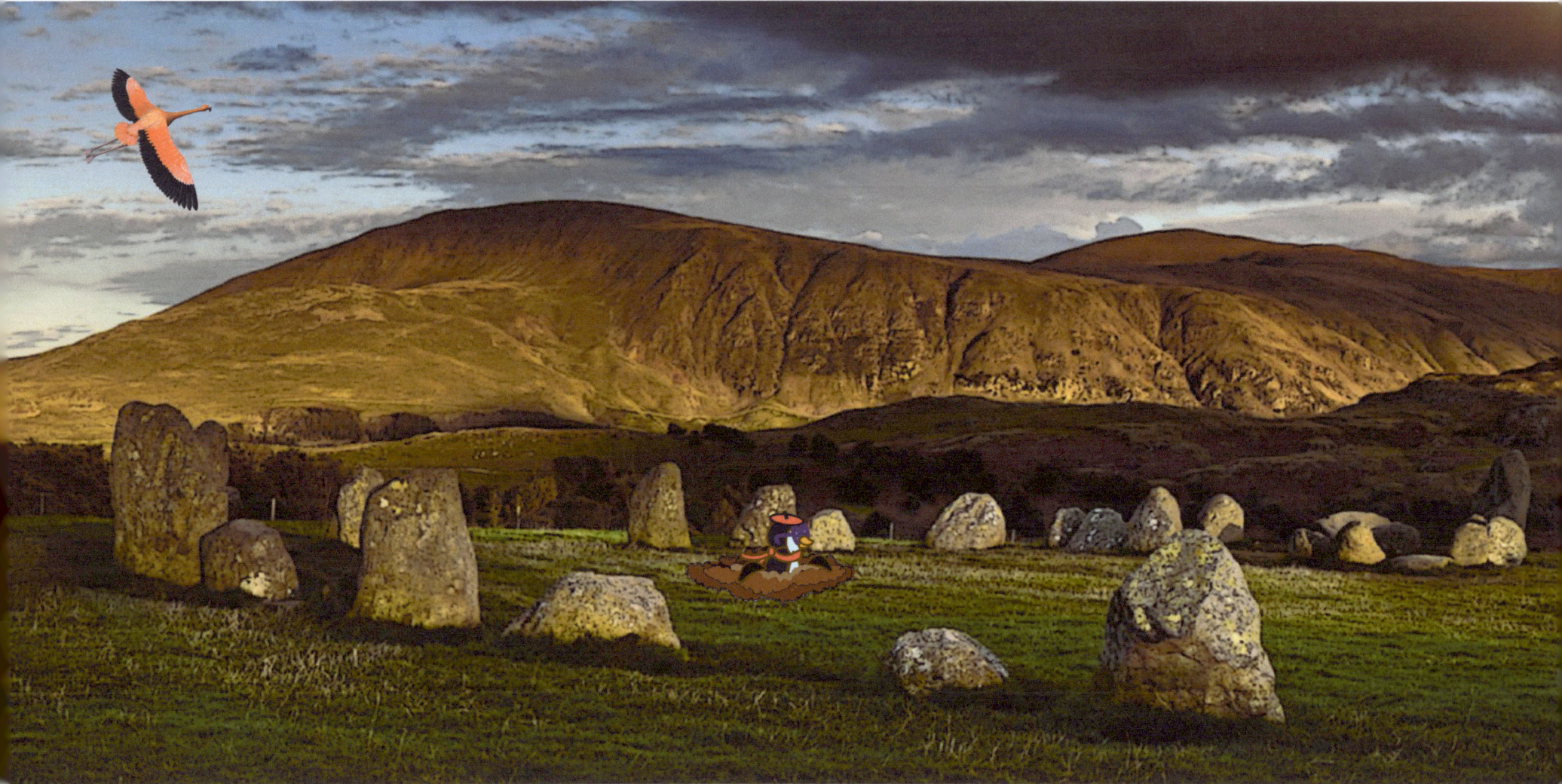

It helps if you sit on something for this posture;
a folded towel, a pillow, your flip flops etc. just something that raises your pelvis off the ground a few centimetres.
4 – 8 cms is good.

Cross your legs and come to a comfortable seated position. Think about making your spine straight. Lift up in the chest,   shoulders back, lift up from the top of your head, dip your chin down a little to make the back of the neck straight then breathe. Relax into the posture and keep your chest up and open. As you exhale feel your shoulder blades slide down your back.

Castlerigg Stone Circle, Keswick, England

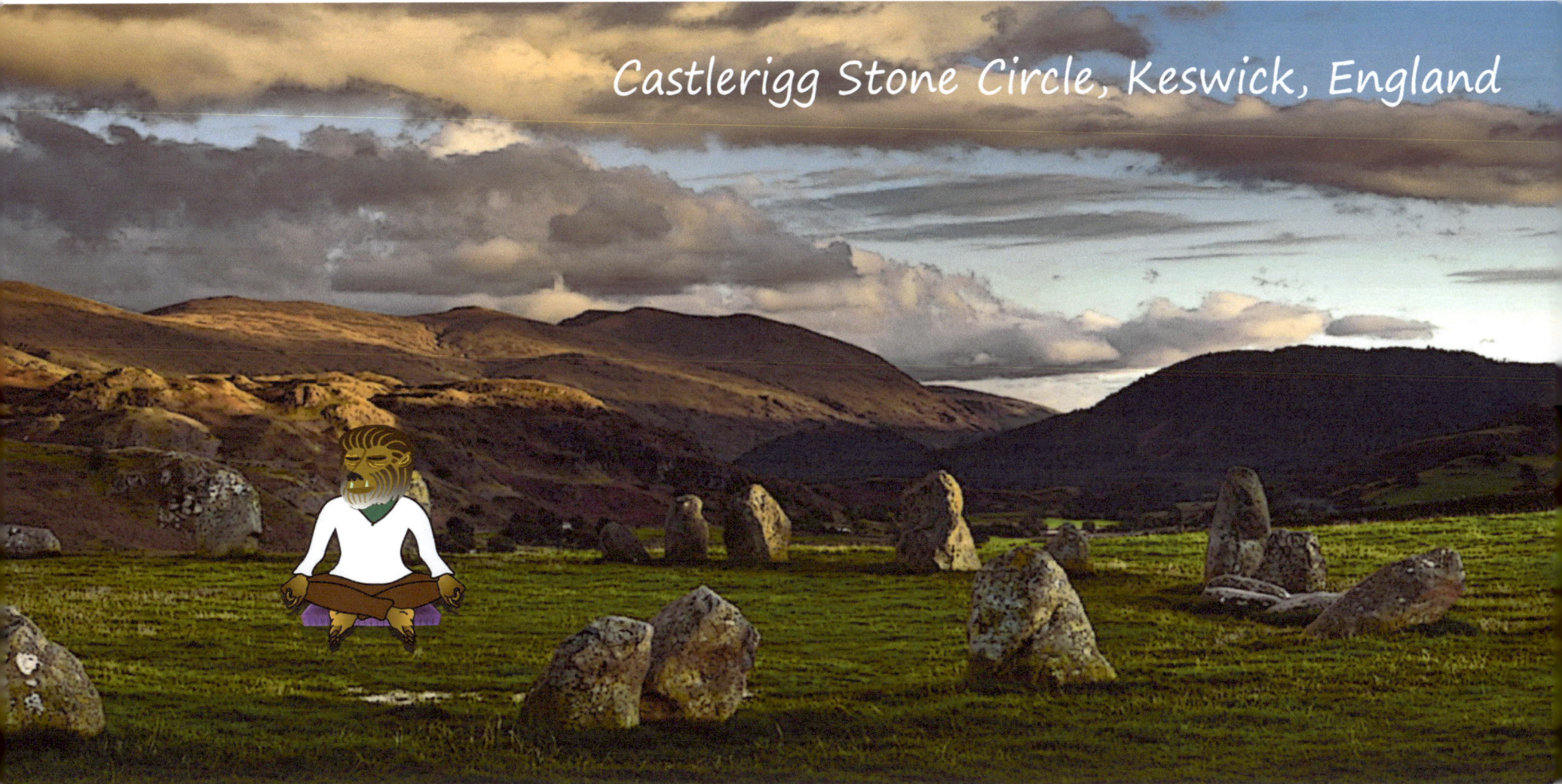

Rest your hands on your knees with the palms facing up and bring the index finger and thumb together, the hands are soft and relaxed. This and other hand positions are called mudra. Take another breath, as you exhale keep the skeleton upright and erect but let your muscles soften and sink down towards the ground. This is Sukhasana; a comfortable seated position and a great posture for meditation.

Meditation

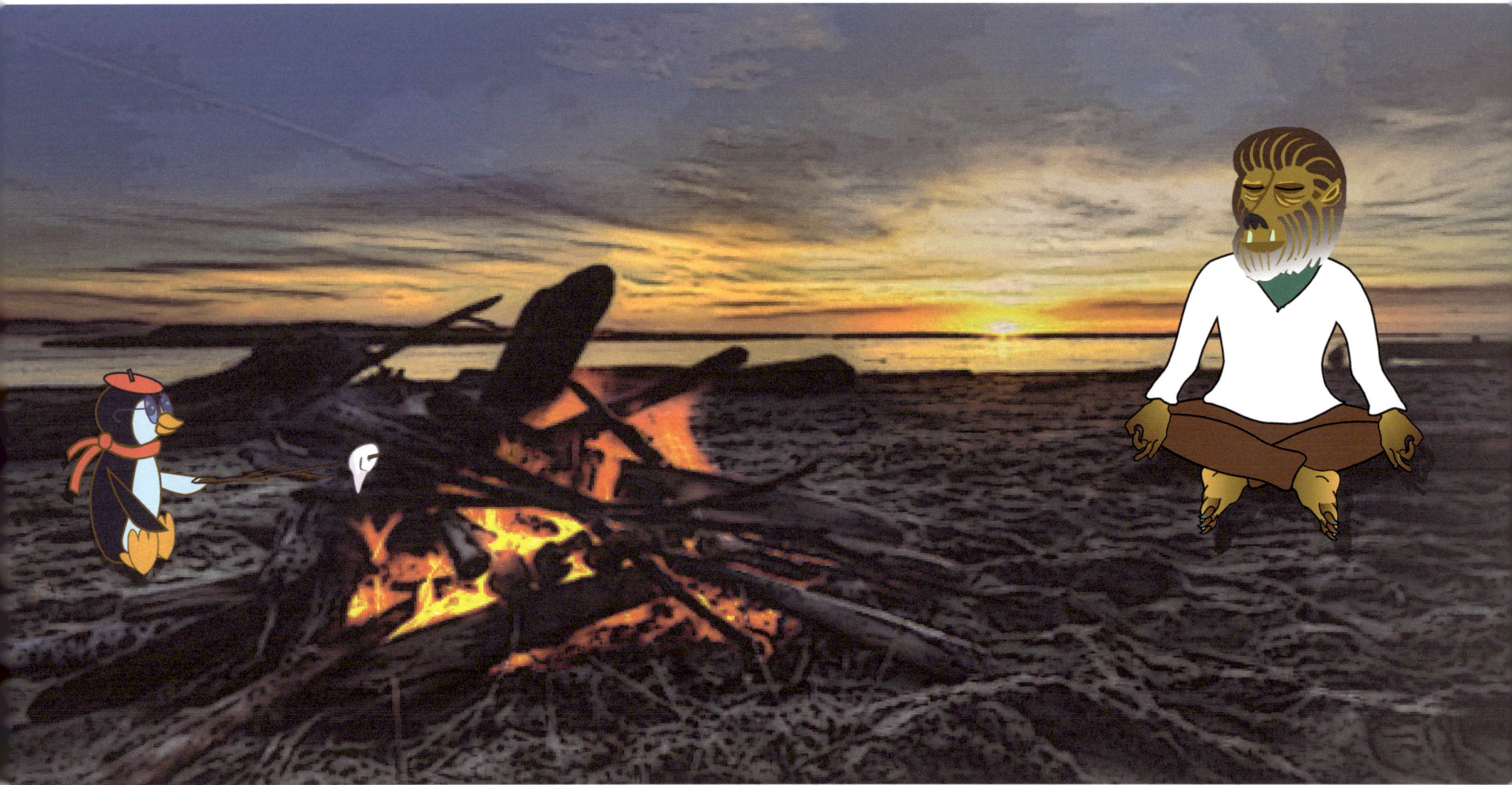

Meditation means to sit quietly and focus your mind on one thing, just like daydreaming. The beauty is that you already do this many times every day. As we learnt before, by focusing the mind we can enhance the effects of any activity we do and meditation is no different. Easy things to meditate on are; your breath, your heart beat, a flower, a candle, a picture or a mandala (see back cover for the Sri Yantra). The great sage Patanjali suggests we can meditate on anything that is elevating to your mind.

For this exercise we will focus on our breath...

Become aware of your spine, think about making it nice and straight. Bring your attention to the tip of your nose and notice the air flow in and out. Follow the breath down into your belly. Inhale belly expands, lungs fill with air, exhale belly contracts pushing the air out of the lungs. Think of the belly like a balloon, inflating and deflating. Take another breath, as you exhale keep your skeleton upright and erect but let your muscles soften and sink down towards the ground. Take ten more breaths like this. Think about making your breath slow, smooth and slender. The inhale is the same length as the exhale. We'll begin to count our breath.

Inhale, 2, 3, 4, Exhale 6, 7, 8. If your mind wanders, bring it back to the counting of the breath.

Inhale, 2, 3, 4, Exhale 6, 7, 8. We'll extend our exhale now to be twice as long as the inhale.

Inhale, 2, 3, 4, Exhale 6, 7, 8, 9, 10, 11, 12.

With each exhalation your mind becomes quiet and your body relaxes. Inhale, 2, 3, 4, Exhale 6, 7, 8, 9, 10, 11, 12.

When the exhale is longer than the inhale you lead more carbon dioxide or waste products out of your body. Your heart rate slows down and you relax. Think about all of the nasty toxins being expelled from your body; the fears, the anxieties, the grief, the worry and the anger. We simply breathe them all away. As you inhale think about the fresh clean oxygen flowing into your body to refresh and rejuvenate your system with prana (life force).

Inhale, 2, 3, 4, Exhale 6, 7, 8, 9, 10, 11, 12. When your mind wanders, bring it back to the counting of the breath.

Inhale, 2, 3, 4, Exhale 6, 7, 8, 9, 10, 11, 12.

Each time the mind wanders you actively bring it back to focus on the task at hand. This helps to train your mind. If you don't train your mind it will run and jump all over the place like a naughty monkey. Then you have to clean up the mess it creates. This technique of training your mind is the basis of all meditation.

As you practice more, day after day, week after week, year after year your mind will become deep and clear. After two or three years you will have trained your mind to be quiet and your body to breath properly. These achievements are not easy, they take time. You have to practice regularly. The more you   practice the easier it gets and the greater the results are. In a while you will come to understand just what a beautiful gift this is; a quiet mind and a full breath.

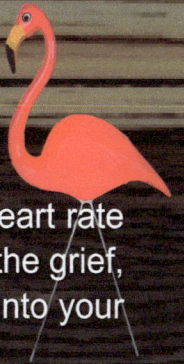

Visualisation

The power of the mind in your yogic practice is very important and helps to enhance the effects of your movements. As I stated before there are many things you can think about during your practice. Imagining colours is an easy place to start. One of the best visuals I recommend is the golden light ball.

If you return now to your breathing;
Inhale, 2, 3, 4, Exhale 6, 7, 8, 9, 10, 11, 12. Keep your spine nice and straight.
Inhale, 2, 3, 4, Exhale 6, 7, 8, 9, 10, 11, 12. Relax your whole body.
Imagine a rising sun inside your belly. As you inhale the sun rises more. Think of this beautiful golden light growing inside you. The more you inhale the more the sun rises, it gets brighter and warmer. With each inhalation the sunshine grows inside of your body. As you exhale breathe out any toxins and negativity. Inhale and feel the sunshine expand within you, growing bigger and bigger. Feel the brilliant golden light fill up your whole body with warmth and happiness, so much so that there is no room left for any darkness and negativity. Breathe out any remaining toxins and smile to yourself. Smile into the sunshine, the warmth, the happiness and the love you created for your self. Take a moment to enjoy the sensations that arise.

Next relax your breathing and let the visuals go. Just let your breathing return to its natural flow. Keep your mind quiet and listening. Notice any sensations that arise be they good or bad, don't give them any attention just notice them, then let them drift away with the breath. Spend a few moments here to enjoy the state of peace and serenity throughout your body. This is called your yoga space or yogic state of mind. It really is a beautiful place to be. Take a moment to smile to yourself and understand that you came here by yourself. I talked and led you here but you followed and actively participated. Now you get to feel the way you do; calm and peaceful. Smile to yourself and enjoy the bliss.

If you came here once, you can do it again, it's really easy if you try. Practice coming here often. There are more than 1000 minutes in a day. Most of this time is given to other people; friends, work, children, television, internet, coffee etc. We forget to take some time for ourselves. If you notice how you feel now, then you will understand it is worth taking a few minutes every day for yourself, so you can be a better person for the people you love. Just five minutes a day will be a great start.

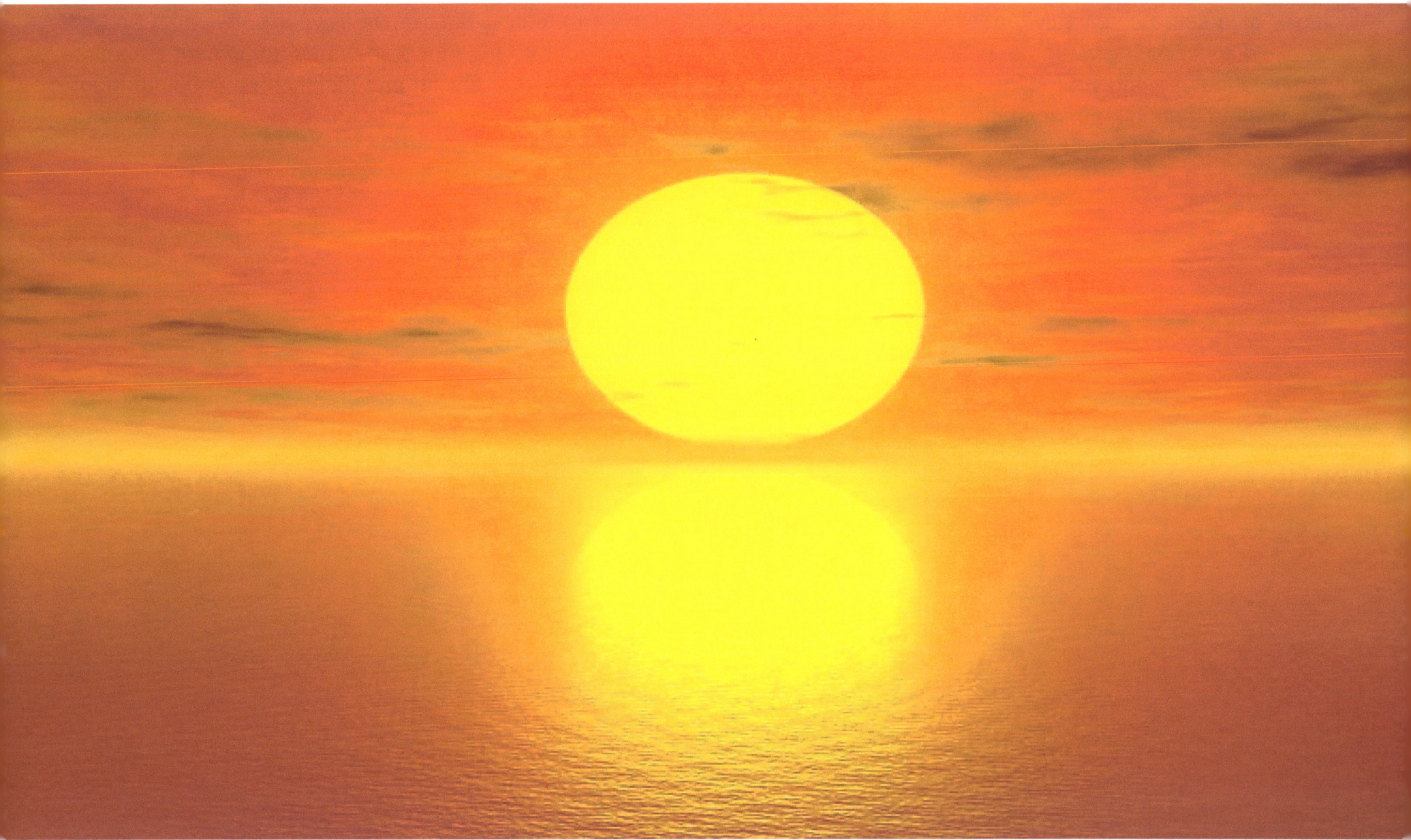

OM

Let's give some chanting/vibration a try. This creates a beautiful warm feeling right down in your gutty wutts and it's really easy to do. All you have to do is hum. The only difference is that it's a long monotone huuuuuuuummmmmmmmmm. Think about making your spine straight but still soft and relaxed. Take a deep breath and simply huuuuuuuuuuuuummmmmmmmmmmmmmmmm! Try this again 5 times. Try to make the lowest sound you can. It doesn't have to be loud, just a low vibraty feeling. Huuuuuuuuuummmmmmmmmmm.

Now try adding another letter to your mmmmmmm sound. The sound 'o', but we make it long just like the mmmmmm.
First oooooooooooooooo, then close the mouth and mmmmmmmmmmmmmmmmm.
Try it again. Take a deep breath and ooooooooooooooooooooooooooommmmmmmmmmmmmmm.
Try it another 5 times. Relax into the sound and let the vibration resonate throughout your whole body.
oooooooooooooooooooooooooooommmmmmmmmmmmmmmmmmmmmmmm.
Smile to yourself and enjoy the sensation of Om vibrating inside you.

Om is the primordial sound of creation, the language of the gods. When god speaks this is what it feels like. Chant it to yourself many times a day to remind you of your divine roots. When you've finished just let the vibration settle down, notice how it feels. It's a really beautiful sensation.

Don't worry about what other people think. When you think of others you break the awesome connection you created for yourself. If this happens then the humming doesn't work properly. So stay focused on what you're doing. Ooooooooooooooooooooooommmmmmmmmmmmmmmmmmmm!

Namaste

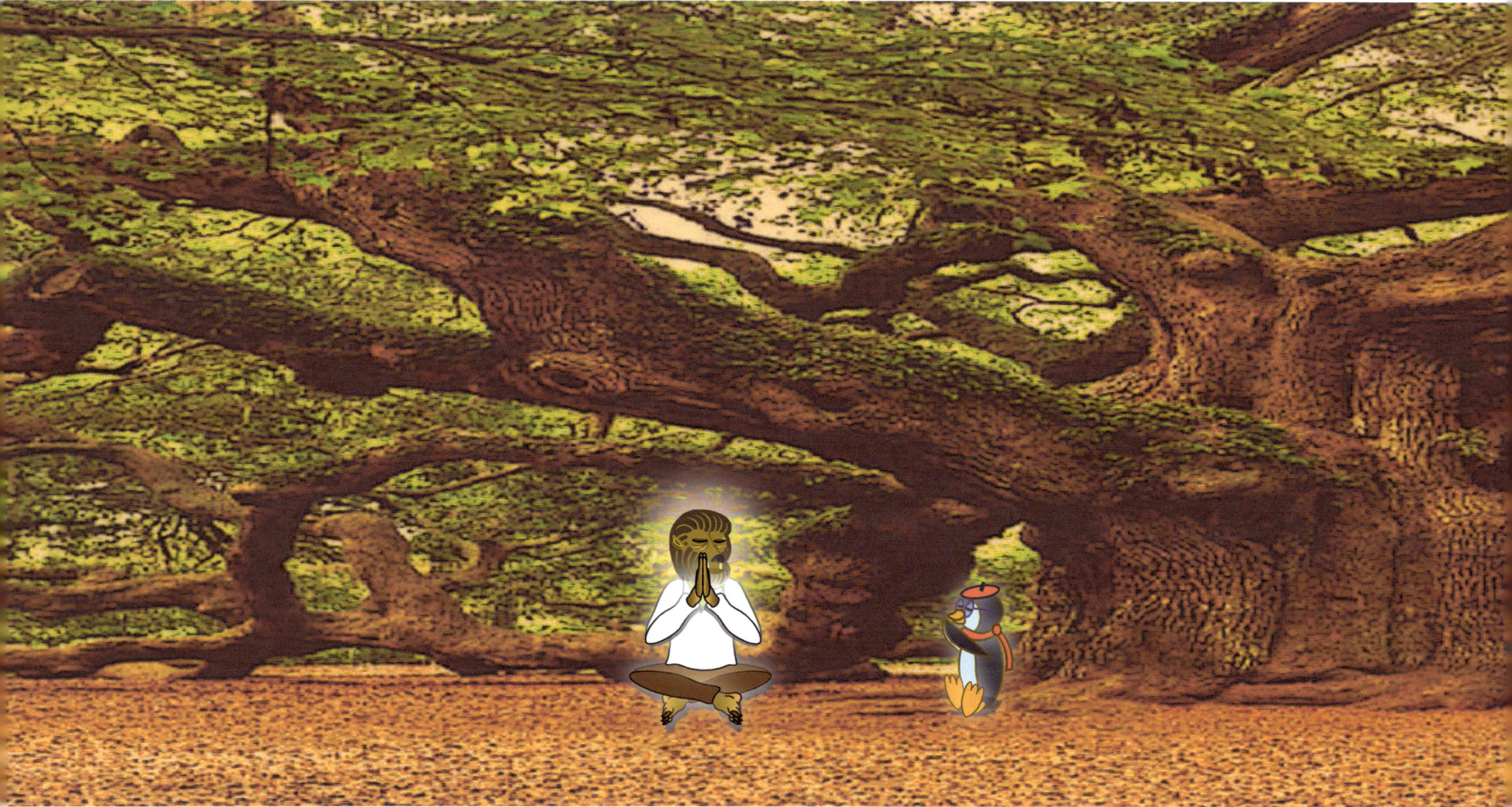

At this point bring your hands together in a prayer position in front of your chest and slightly bow the head. This position is called Anjali Mudra. Close your eyes and give thanks to the masters and teachers who have gone down the path of yoga before you. Acknowledge each other for keeping these practices alive and smile to yourself.

Then we say Namaste (na-mas-tay).

Namaste means the goodness and divine in me, respects the goodness and divine in you. So namaste friends! Stretch out your legs and give them a good shake. If you are new to these practices, then your body probably isn't used to sitting still and will tense up a little. This is normal. Tap your legs and shake them to get the blood flowing normally again. Remember to smile and enjoy the sensations your body creates.

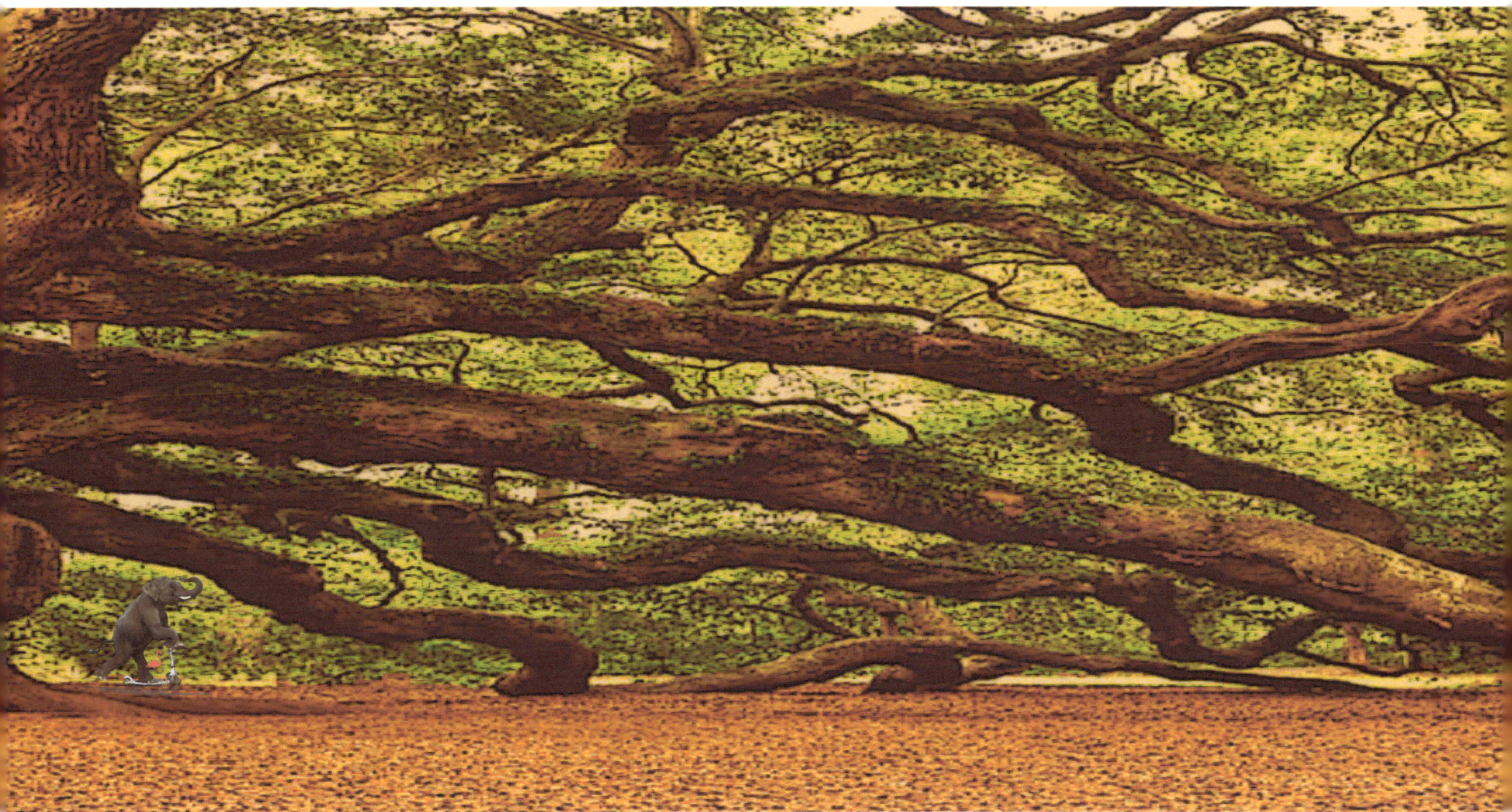

I trust you feel great and I hope you've learned something. Take the time to practice a little each day, five minutes is a great start. Thanks for being a part of this wonderful session and have an awesome day.
I look forward to our next adventure together.

What's next?

Yoga is something you incorporate into your life, it becomes a thing you do every day. Like a cup of coffee, or brushing your teeth, going to the toilet, sleeping or even talking. When this happens you begin to find the balance that yoga gives. As I said before advanced yogic techniques may not be for everybody, but basic practices that you can use every day will be of great benefit. The asanas and movements I've outlined in this book are enough to keep you feeling good, happy and balanced for the rest of your life, if you use them.

The best time for yoga is in the morning or in the evening, or when you yawn and stretch. This is your body's way of asking to be opened, please help me it says. Other times are when you have nothing to do or have some time to kill. Say you're waiting for a friend and they will be another ten minutes, that's the time to practice a few simple moves. Then when your friend arrives you will be happier and ready to embrace your friendship. It doesn't matter which moves you do; the mountain pose, big breaths, lifting a ball, floppy twist, forward bend, cheeky monkey, cap on the top, hip circles, tapping, visualisation or just quiet breathing. What matters are the moments you take to connect with your body!

If you're interested in studying further, then physically the next phase is called Surya Namaskar, The Sun Salutation. This practice seeks to strengthen and develop your spine. After this comes the 12 basic postures of hatha yoga. Hatha means sun and moon, and seeks to find the balance between these two energies and how they relate to the body. In China they're called Yin and Yang. In regard to text, I'd recommend Patanjali's Yoga Sutras, The Upanishads, The Bhagavad Gita, The Dhammapada and The Tao Te Ching. These books were written in other languages so it's important to find a good translation. They will keep you busy for many, many years of study. In spiritual advancement it's important to steer clear of religion and stick to philosophy. Yoga, Buddhism and Taoism are philosophies, not religion. They promote a way of being not dogmatic servitude.

It is advised to seek a good teacher to help you on your way whichever path you may choose. Who is the right teacher? Only you can answer that. But as they say in the scriptures; when the student is ready the teacher will appear. If you seek, you will find the answers to all of your questions. The key is persistence. The road ahead is not an easy one but if you keep striving for truth you will get there. Ultimately yoga is a movement towards the divine source or God. If you keep knocking on the door of spirituality, one day God himself will open it and invite you in.

Baruch Hashem

Yangshuo, China

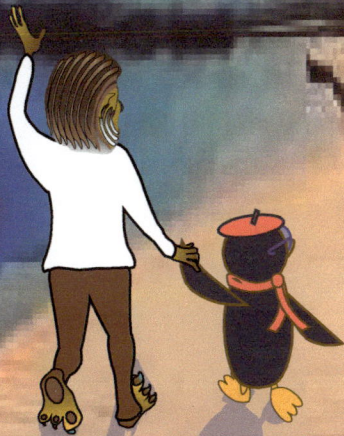

When you move amidst the world of sense, free from attachment and aversion alike, there comes the peace in which all sorrows end, and you live in the wisdom of the Self.

Bhagavad Gita.

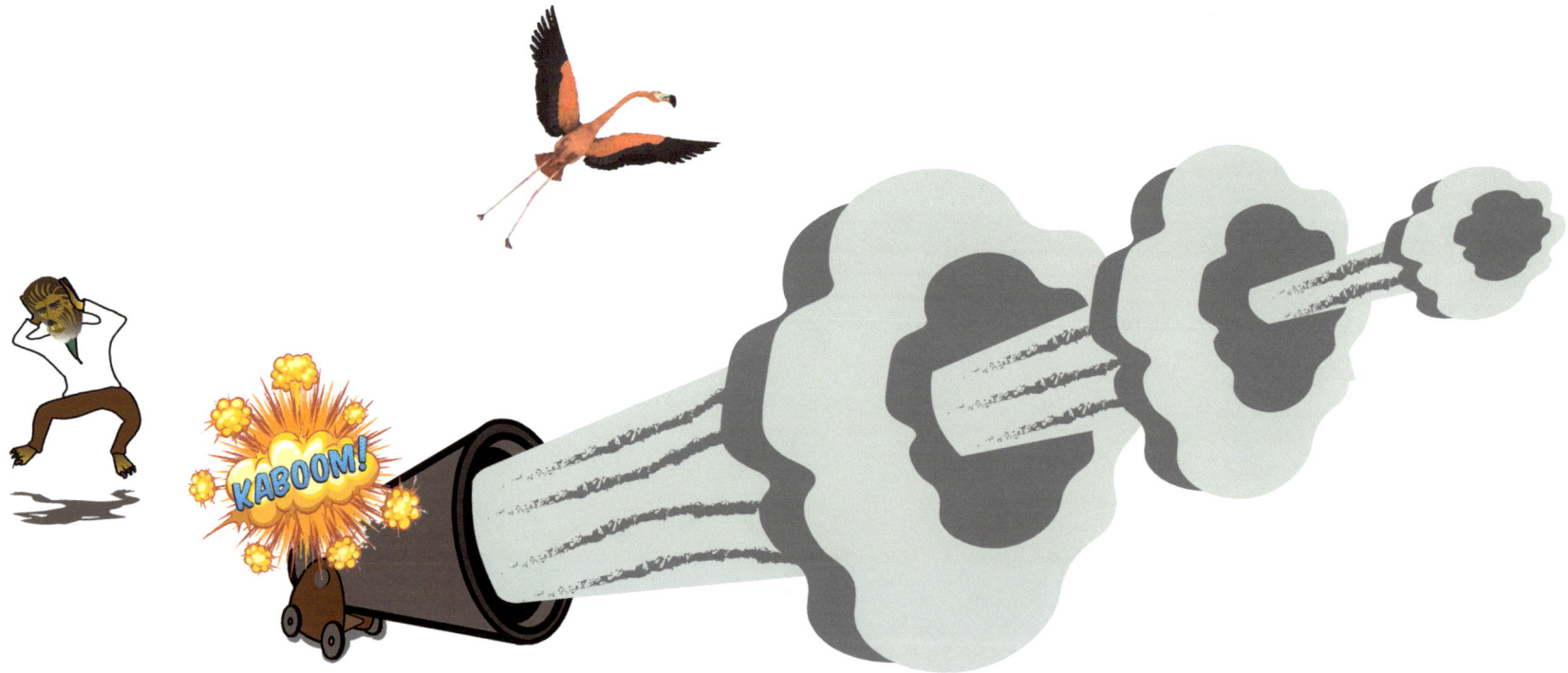

Hint – The back cover is a 10,000 year old sacred geometrical tool. It's called Sri Yantra. Take some time to watch it. Surrender your mind to the shapes and the lines. Look deep into the image. If you meditate long enough you might see it move ;)

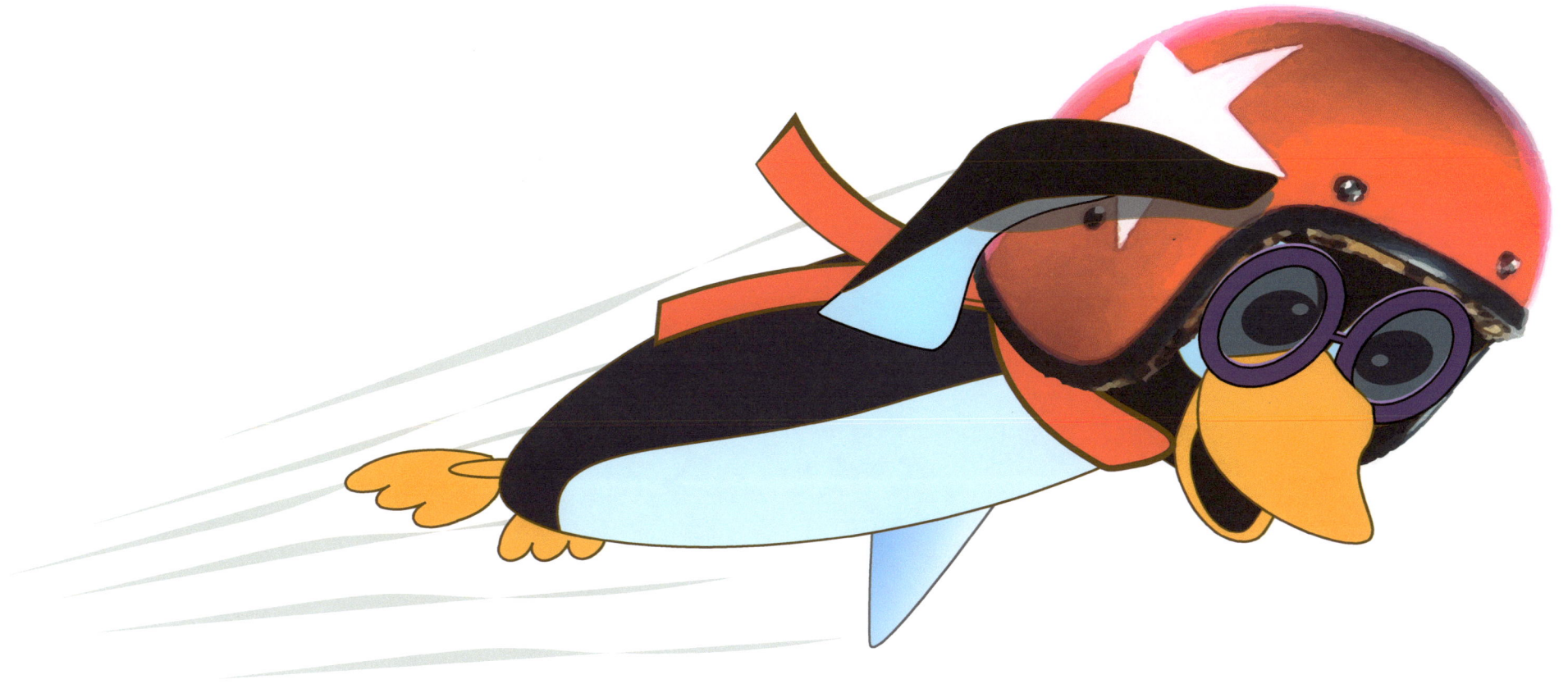

Bon Voyage!

www.ingramcontent.com/pod-product-compliance
Lightning Source LLC
Chambersburg PA
CBHW041549030426

42334CB00006B/104